the
mediterrasian
way

the
mediterrasian
way

A COOKBOOK AND GUIDE TO HEALTH, WEIGHT LOSS,
AND LONGEVITY, COMBINING THE BEST FEATURES OF
MEDITERRANEAN AND ASIAN DIETS AND LIFESTYLES

Ric Watson
and Trudy Thelander

BICENTENNIAL
1807
WILEY
2007
BICENTENNIAL

JOHN WILEY & SONS, INC.

Library of Congress Cataloging-in-Publication Data

Watson, Ric.
     The MediterrAsian way / by Ric Watson and Trudy Thelander.
        p. cm.
     Includes bibliographical references and index.
     ISBN 978-0-470-04558-9 (cloth)
  1. Nutrition. 2. Diet--Mediterranean Region. 3. Diet--Asia. 4. Cookery, Mediterranean. 5. Cookery, Asian. I. Thelander, Trudy. II. Title.

  RA784.W423 2007
  641.595--dc22

                              2006016600

Printed in the United States of America

10 9 8 7 6 5 4 3 2 1

INTERIOR DESIGN: DEBORAH KERNER DESIGN
COVER DESIGN: SUZANNE SUNWOO
WILEY BICENTENNIAL LOGO DESIGN: RICHARD J. PACIFICO

Contents

RECIPES *141*

ACKNOWLEDGMENTS

We'd like to start by thanking the many scientists, doctors, and dieticians who have devoted their time to researching traditional Mediterranean and Asian dietary and lifestyle practices. Without the pioneering work of people such as Professor Ancel Keys and Dr. T. Colin Campbell the many health-giving benefits of this way of living would never have come to light in the first place.

Thanks to all the people who have sent e-mails to MediterrAsian.com offering us words of encouragement and support. We hope the information and recipes in this book make it even easier for you to incorporate traditional Mediterranean and Asian practices into your own life.

We're very grateful to our agent, Stacey Glick, for helping us put our ideas into print and for guiding us through the world of publishing.

The hard-working team at Wiley deserve a big thank you. Especially our editor Justin Schwartz, and also Ava Wilder, Deborah Kerner, Christine DiComo, Jacqueline Beach, and Christina Solazzo.

Thanks to our families for giving us love and encouragement. Thanks also to family members who helped shape our lives but who are no longer with us—in particular Ric's dad, Richard.

Finally, thanks to Oldways Preservation and Exchange Trust for kindly granting us permission to use the Mediterranean and Asian Diet Pyramids in this book.

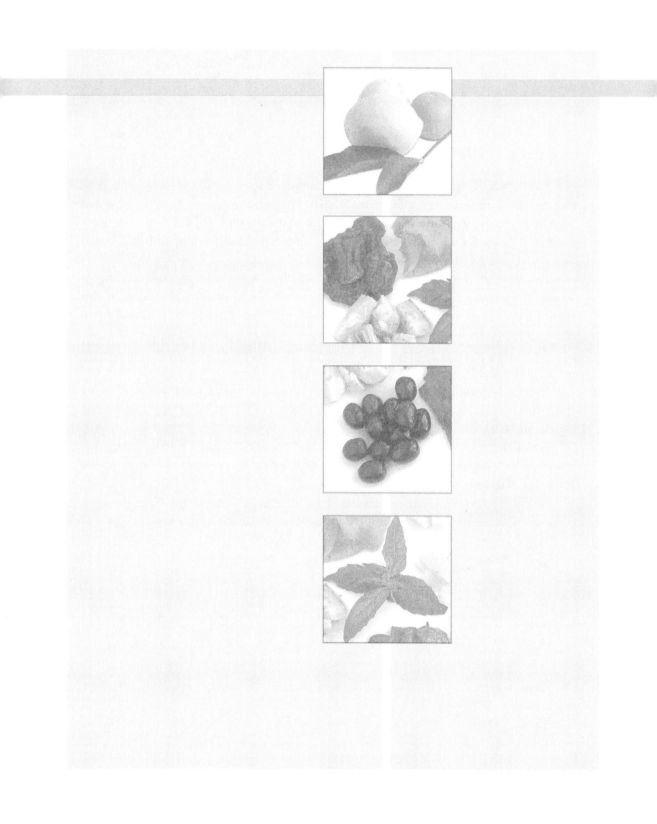

the mediterrasian way

I believe that by following Mediterranean and Asian dietary and lifestyle practices you can change your health, and your life, for the better. And I don't make that statement lightly. I know firsthand the benefits of this way of living, because it's had a very dramatic impact on my life. So, before describing this lifestyle in detail and how it can change your life, I'd like to tell you a little bit about myself and how a MediterrAsian lifestyle has changed my own life.

LIFE LESSONS

I was born to English parents in the beautiful Pacific Island nation of New Zealand. My parents had migrated to New Zealand because my dad, who was serving in the British Royal Airforce, had received a transfer there. And from as far back as I can remember, I'd dreamed of following in his footsteps by joining the military. But unlike my dad, who served in the air force, I planned on becoming an officer in the army.

When I was a child, everything seemed to be heading in the right direction. I was very physically active when I was young and loved sports. I was lucky enough in my school days to be selected to play representative rugby for my city. One year I also set a school record in the 200-meter sprint. So, as far as I was concerned, I was well prepared for a physically demanding career as a soldier.

But, as the old saying goes, *the best-laid plans often go astray.*

First, in 1984, I was called out of art class at school to the principal's office. My mother greeted me in tears and told me that my dad, who suffered from bouts of severe depression, had taken his own life.

Then, less than a year later—and while I was still grieving my dad's death—I was involved in a high-speed collision with a car while I was riding my motorcycle to a friend's house. My unprotected body slammed into the hard metal chassis with so much force that I broke most of the major bones on the left side my body. My left kneecap was shattered into several pieces, I sustained multiple lacerations, I severely bruised my liver and kidneys, and I lost a great deal of blood.

After being laid up for two months in the hospital, I was left with what my orthopedic surgeon described as "a permanent left-sided disability." And he told me that I might even need to use a walking stick for the rest of my life. He also told me flatly, but honestly, that I had "very little chance" of ever becoming a soldier.

These two horrible events, particularly one coming so soon after the other, took a toll on me, both physically and emotionally. But I'd already learned from my dad's death that you can't dwell on a crisis. You somehow have to see a positive (no matter how small that positive may be) and move on, or else it will just eat you up.

I started to look for positives and thought about how my surgeon had given me very little chance of becoming a soldier, but he hadn't said "no chance at all." As far as I was concerned, even if there was less than a 1 percent chance, I was still willing to give it a go. I knew I had nothing to lose.

A SEARCH FOR ANSWERS

So I decided to look for ways to regain my health and become fit and strong again. As Napoleon Bonaparte once said, "There are two ways to move men—interest and fear," and I certainly had both! Unfortunately, what I didn't have was any idea how to regain my health once it had been lost. I came to the conclusion that I needed to learn all I could about diet, health, and fitness if I was ever going to have a chance of reclaiming my future.

The first places I turned to for answers were bookstores and libraries. I was pleasantly surprised to find the shelves virtually overflowing with books promising a fast route to good health. However, on closer inspection, I noticed that most of these books offered different solutions from one another. In a lot of cases, one expert would totally contradict what another equally well-qualified expert said. I was staggered by the number of mixed messages I found.

In desperation I was forced to try a lot of different ways to regain my health. I found most of them were very restrictive, and the results were mostly disappointing. But I persevered, because I realized that my entire future was on the line.

Eventually, after more than a year of *hard* work, I'd reached a point where I felt I could give the army a go. My knee was still causing me a lot of pain, and I knew I certainly wasn't back to 100 percent health, but I figured that army life would somehow "whip me into shape." In the end, I knew it was going to be a struggle, but I was determined to grit my teeth and face the challenge.

However, although I was mentally prepared, physically my body certainly wasn't. By the end of the first day of training my knee started to swell and became increasingly painful. By the end of the week my knee was the size of a small balloon, and the pain was almost unbearable. I begged the army physician to let me stay to see if it improved, but he realized there was just no chance. So, after only eight days, I was honorably discharged from the army.

I returned home feeling like a failure. I couldn't believe that more than a year of struggle and sacrifice had amounted to absolutely nothing. But I knew I'd come too far to quit. I was still positive that the answer to regaining my health was out there somewhere, and at this stage I was more determined than ever to find it.

Again, I went back to the books and tried a number of other "miracle breakthroughs." Eventually, after four months of resolute effort, I felt I could give the army another go. It took a great deal of work to convince the army physician that I was fit and strong enough to reenlist, but after fervently pleading my case, he gave the go-ahead. I was over the moon. I couldn't believe I'd been given a second chance.

But my happiness quickly turned to despair when, after only a day of training, the swelling and pain in my knee started to increase. I tried lots of ways of covering up the pain and inflammation, but when my pants wouldn't fit over my knee anymore, I knew I was fighting a losing battle. So, after a little over a week back in the army, I received my second honorable discharge.

I returned home in a worse state than ever—both physically and emotionally. My orthopedic surgeon's report from the time highlights the poor state of my physical health:

> The wrist is painful . . . his left leg is troublesome and in particular the knee. Strenuous activity causes pain, standing causes the knee to ache and swell, he can jog for a mile but then has considerable pain which is quite persistent. He cannot run, cannot kneel, has difficulty getting up and down stairs . . . and the knee causes quite severe episodic pain.

The report finished on a high note: *"The situation is unlikely to change."*

I was devastated. And at this point I was well and truly fed up with what life had thrown at me: my dad's suicide, my accident, in and out of the army twice. Trying everything in my power to regain my health, yet being in a worse state of health and in more pain than ever. As far as I was concerned, I was just destined to be a shell of my former self—one of life's "unlucky" people.

As 1987 drew to a close, the outlook for my future seemed very bleak indeed. However, just as I was hitting rock bottom, something unexpected happened. I discovered that an accident compensation claim I'd filed many months earlier had been settled, and I'd received a lump-sum payment of $13,000.

Back in the '80s—and to a young, single guy down on his luck—$13,000 dollars seemed like a small fortune! But at first I wasn't quite sure what to do with it. Like most young guys, thoughts of fast cars, new clothes, and expansion of my music collection all came to mind. But I knew there was a much deeper significance to getting this money. I knew it was the only ray of hope I had left for improving my future, and I was determined to use it very wisely.

One thing I knew for certain, I needed a break—a *big* break. My stress levels were going through the roof, and the severe pain in my left knee was really getting me down. I was also out of shape because my knee prevented me from being physically active. I knew a long holiday would help me recuperate.

It didn't take me long to decide on the south coast of England as my holiday destination. Not just because of the peacefulness of this area, but because my uncle Tony lived there. And in many ways, Tony was the last hope I had for regaining my health.

THE HOLIDAY THAT CHANGED MY LIFE

Tony, like my father, had served in the British Royal Airforce. But, instead of transferring to New Zealand, Tony had been stationed in the Middle East (where they traditionally eat a Mediterranean-style diet). It was there during the 1960s that Tony became a middleweight boxing champion for the air force. When Tony returned to England he left the air force. During the '70s and '80s, he was a sports coach and ran his own gymnasium.

When I arrived in England in early 1988, Tony and his wife, Muriel, were living in a quiet country village near the sea where they were running their own health spa. At the time Tony was in his late forties, but I was taken aback when I first saw him—he was in extraordinary physical condition and didn't look a day over thirty-five. Even more surprising was Aunt Muriel, who was nearly ten years older than Tony and approaching sixty. I could only describe her as radiant, and I would have sworn she wouldn't be blowing out more than forty candles on her next birthday. It was immediately clear that these people knew more than a few secrets about getting and staying fit and healthy, and I was determined to pick their brains!

One of my biggest surprises was when I discovered just how much good food Tony and Muriel ate. It turned out that the time Tony had spent stationed overseas had had a big influence on him, and there were no carrot sticks or servings of cottage cheese anywhere in sight. Instead, I found delicious and hearty pasta, bean, vegetable, and rice dishes; a wide range of breads and cheeses; eggs; nuts; olive oil; seasonal and tropical fruits; and wonderful desserts.

Tony also told me that he and Muriel hadn't eaten red meat for years. He said that small amounts of red meat were fine but that I should preferably eat chicken or, better still, fish and shellfish, which he said contained special health-giving oils. Tony also explained that eating the correct balance of these foods was just as important as the food itself.

At first it seemed almost too good to be true that by eating these delicious foods I could get healthy and in shape. But as soon as I started eating the correct balance of the foods Tony recommended, I could feel my body absorb the concentrated nourishment like a dry sponge soaking up water. Within days my energy level had increased substantially. Within weeks the pain and inflammation around my knee had started to improve noticeably. Even the excess weight I'd gained from my lack of movement started dropping off. And to my delight I discovered there was another positive side effect. Since I was six years old I'd suffered from migraine headaches almost weekly. My parents had taken me to a number of medical specialists in search of a cure, without success. But these nausea-inducing headaches that had plagued me most of my life simply disappeared.

I'd heard that "you are what you eat," but I was amazed that something as simple as making the right food choices could have such a dramatic effect on my health. In fact, within six months my strength and energy had improved so much that I was even able to run for long distances, with only a minimum of discomfort.

After so much time fruitlessly struggling to regain my health, I could hardly believe the remarkable improvement in my health, fitness, and energy in such a short amount of time. A few months earlier I could barely walk up a flight of stairs, and running for any distance caused almost unbearable pain. Yet here I was, running for miles at a time with virtually no pain. My energy levels were at an all-time high, I was free of migraine headaches, and I was more than twenty pounds lighter. As far as I was concerned, it was nothing short of a miracle!

MOVING ON

With such a positive outcome, my holiday to England, which I'd originally planned to last no longer than two months, ended up turning into a working vacation lasting more than a year. But eventually I realized that although I'd sorted out my health, I was still single and without a career. I knew it was time to move on.

Instead of immediately returning home to New Zealand, I decided to visit my mother, who had remarried and moved to Australia. As it turned out, this was one of the most fateful decisions I've ever made, because it was in Australia that I met and fell in love with the coauthor of this book, Trudy.

PERFECT MATCH

When I first met Trudy I couldn't believe how much we had in common. Like me, she was very interested in looking after her health (I found out that this was because she was the daughter of two practicing medical doctors). She also loved traveling (so much so that she was an international travel agent), and just like me she loved good food, good wine, and good conversation. With such an incentive to stay in Australia, I decided to indefinitely postpone my return to New Zealand, and Trudy and I moved in together.

With our common passion for good food, it wasn't long before we found ourselves naturally gravitating toward the kitchen. I was particularly keen to introduce Trudy to all the wonderful and healthy Mediterranean-style dishes I'd learned to cook in England. And I discovered that Trudy was equally keen to introduce me to her favorite style of food: Asian. It turned out that Trudy's sister-in-law was Chinese Malaysian and had introduced her to authentic Asian cooking years earlier; Trudy had been hooked ever since. And as soon as I tasted my first mouthful of the authentic Asian seafood stir-fry that Trudy whipped up, I was well and truly hooked, too!

At first I was worried about deviating too much from the Mediterranean style of eating I had been following. I thought that if I ate too much Asian-inspired food, the pain in my knee could flare up, and my migraine headaches might return. Yet the more I looked into it the more I realized that, apart from basic differences in herbs and flavorings, the diets of the Mediterranean and Asia were actually remarkably similar.

For example, the traditional focal point of a meal in both Mediterranean and Asian cultures is a grain food. In Asia it's rice and noodles, and in the Mediterranean it's pasta, rice, bread, and other grain foods, such as couscous and bulgur. And red meats don't feature prominently in either cuisine; instead fish, shellfish, poultry, and plant foods such as beans and nuts form the main sources of protein. Asian and Mediterranean peoples also traditionally eat lots of fresh vegetables and fruits, and even the type of fat they use is similar, favoring healthy vegetable fats such as olive or peanut oil over animal fats. Finally, the consumption of moderate amounts of alcohol, particularly over a meal, has been practiced by Mediterranean and Asian cultures for centuries. So, although each type of cuisine is unique, the nutrients found in both the Mediterranean- and Asian-style diets are practically identical. This delighted me because it opened up a whole new world of tastes and textures without compromising my hard-won good health. In fact, this way of eating made so much sense that it wasn't long before Trudy and I were living on an almost exclusive diet of what we called "MediterrAsian" food—literally, a fusion of Mediterranean and Asian cuisines.

GOOD FOOD THAT'S GOOD FOR YOU

As we experimented more and more with a MediterrAsian style of eating, we were delighted to discover that, in addition to all the health benefits, there were countless other bonuses too. For one, it never ceased to amaze us that foods this healthful were also the most delicious we'd ever tasted. And, as we began to experiment more with fresh Mediterranean and Asian ingredients, we found that the healthiest way to cook them was often the simplest, which meant less work for the cook! Best of all, this way of eating offered us such an endless variety of unique tastes, intriguing textures, vibrant colors, and tantalizing aromas that we were never bored. In fact, far from restricting our choice, we discovered a world of diverse foods and flavors.

To our delight, we also discovered that most of our favorite restaurant and takeout food was based on the cuisines of the Mediterranean and Asia. Italian, Greek, Indian, Chinese, French Provençal, Japanese, Thai, Vietnamese, Turkish, Spanish, Moroccan, and Lebanese were just some of the ethnic delights we could choose from.

With our love for this type of food we also became enthusiastic collectors of Mediterranean and Asian recipes. Our search for new and interesting dishes was helped immeasurably by Trudy's job as a travel agent. One of the perks of her job was traveling the world inspecting the facilities of international hotels. She used these overseas trips to such places as Indonesia and Hong Kong as the perfect opportunity to add to our growing collection of recipes. She would always return home with a notebook full of hastily scribbled recipes she had picked up from street vendors or in traditional backstreet eateries—food that was so simple, yet utterly glorious.

However, as appetizing and varied as all this Mediterranean and Asian food was, we found that occasionally we still got cravings for some of our old Western favorites, like cheeseburgers and hot dogs. We knew that because the majority of food we ate was so naturally healthy, the occasional fast-food binge was OK. But by experimenting and using the principles and techniques we'd learned through Mediterranean and Asian cooking, we discovered that we could actually adapt these typically unhealthy foods and create far healthier versions without sacrificing the taste. After a lot of experimentation, we eventually developed, among other things, healthy and tasty versions of hamburgers, hot dogs, fries, and subs.

To us, this was the best of both worlds: the rich culinary diversity of Asia and the Mediterranean region, plus healthy, tasty versions of our old favorites.

DISCOVERING MORE THAN FOOD

Over the years our love of Mediterranean and Asian food became a true passion. But it went a lot deeper than just food. We also became fascinated by the culture and rich history of these areas. And as we'd reaped so many positive rewards simply by adopting this style of eating, we started to wonder whether we could learn other lifestyle lessons from these cultures too.

Our first thoughts turned to our least favorite activity in life: exercising. At this stage, the main form of exercise in our lives was exercise sessions at our local fitness center. We both found this type of exercise extremely boring and a lot of hard work. Including the cost of yearly membership and parking, it was also very expensive. But we were under the impression that it was a necessary evil we just had to put up with if we wanted to stay fit. Then it dawned on us: For the past few thousand years Mediterranean and Asian peoples had never worked out on Stairmasters or Butt-Blasters or jumped around in aerobics classes to stay in shape. They kept fit by simply moving naturally as part of their everyday lives, so why couldn't we do the same?

This thought encouraged us to start looking for ways we could move naturally as part of our everyday lives, instead of moving artificially at the fitness center. We soon discovered dozens of ways we could easily and effortlessly slip physical activity into our lives without formally exercising, and all of them were a lot more fun than sweating away on a Stairmaster. Before long we decided to give up the fitness center and artificial exercise all together.

NOURISHING THE BODY AND THE SOUL

Between the healthy foods we were eating and the natural movement we were incorporating into our lives, we couldn't have been physically healthier. But as important as our physical well-being is, we also know from personal experience that our emotional well-being is just as important.

By adopting a MediterrAsian style of eating, we had discovered how to enjoy lots of wonderful food while staying healthy and in shape, so this certainly went a long way toward providing us with a good sense of emotional well-being. But we knew that eating good food is only one of life's many pleasures. So we began to think of other ways we could achieve emotional well-being in our lives that didn't revolve around food. Through lots of fun experimentation we discovered plenty of ways to relax, rejuvenate, and achieve a sense emotional well-being in our lives, and none of them involved food. (This was good not only for our emotional well-being but for the well-being of our waistlines too!)

We soon made it a rule that every day, no matter how busy we were, we each had to set aside time to do something relaxing and enjoyable. We found that one of the big benefits of having relaxation time every day, apart from recharging our emotional and spiritual batteries, was that it also acted as a very effective stress-reliever.

PUTTING IT ALL TOGETHER

For us, incorporating relaxation time into our lives completed the foundations for achieving a healthy body and mind. And in many ways we had relied on the basic principles that Mediterranean and Asian peoples had instinctively been living for the past few thousand years: We were eating lots of good wholesome food; we were physically active as part of our everyday lives; and, by setting aside special time to relax every day, we were mimicking the relaxed, less stressful lifestyles that characterize people from these regions. With this simple three-pronged approach toward our physical and emotional health, not only did we feel empowered but we ultimately felt we had achieved that most elusive of all states: *optimal health*.

SOLVING THE MYSTERY

Adopting a MediterrAsian way of living had made a profound difference to our health and vitality. Yet, although we knew that this lifestyle worked, we still didn't know exactly *why* it worked. This got us thinking: Was there a scientific explanation for the way we were feeling? Luckily this question became a lot easier to answer in 1996, when we connected our home computer to the most powerful research tool in the world, the Internet.

Suddenly, at our fingertips, we had access to cutting-edge research from some of the world's most respected universities, hospitals, and research centers, including Harvard, Cornell, and Oxford. What we found amazed and enlightened us. Yes, there certainly was a scientific explanation for the way we were feeling. We discovered that for more than half a century some of the Western world's leading scientists and doctors had been thoroughly investigating the health-giving benefits of Mediterranean and Asian dietary and lifestyle practices.

We uncovered hundreds of interviews, reports, articles, and well-documented scientific studies that confirm why this way of living was so beneficial. And, as we investigated deeper, we discovered dozens of remarkable stories of other Westerners, like us, who had adopted a similar lifestyle and were reaping incredible benefits.

Among other things, we found that this type of lifestyle had been credited with the prevention of long-term crippling illnesses such as heart disease, many types of cancer, and arthritis.

SHARING OUR KNOWLEDGE

By 1997 it was hard to believe how dramatically my life had turned around in the years since my accident. From thinking of myself as one of life's unlucky people, I now felt like one of the luckiest people in the world. I was fitter and stronger both physically and emotionally than ever before; I was sharing my life with someone I adored; and, to top it off, I'd even found a career I loved—I'd combined a lifelong passion for art with a computer, and I started my own graphic design business.

But as happy and complete as my life seemed, I couldn't help thinking about how differently things could have turned out. I realized that if it wasn't for an extraordinary set of circumstances I never would have fully regained my health at all. This was reinforced to me every time I saw a new book or infomercial claiming to have finally discovered the "real answer" to getting healthy and fit. I knew most of these so-called answers were simply the same gimmicky personal theories that were around when I was struggling to regain my health back in the '80s, only with slick new packaging and flashy new marketing.

This made me feel incredibly frustrated, because I knew we'd found a real answer: We'd discovered how someone living a busy Western lifestyle could successfully adopt the traditional dietary and lifestyle practices of the healthiest peoples on earth. And this answer wasn't based on someone's personal theory; it was based on dietary and lifestyle practices that had been successfully tried and tested for more than five thousand years.

We were positive there were lots of other people out there, like me, who had lost their health—either through accident, illness, or obesity—who would really appreciate knowing about this way of living. I certainly knew that if this sort of information had been available when I was fruitlessly searching for answers, it would have saved me a huge amount of frustration and emotional anxiety.

So we decided to become proactive. We made up our minds that we were going to share what we knew about this way of living with as many people as we could. But we had one major stumbling block. We had no idea how to get this information out to anybody except our family and friends.

After a lot of deliberation, Trudy suggested that we record a phone message setting out the basic principles of a MediterrAsian way of living, and people could simply phone in and listen to it. This made a lot of sense to me, because it seemed like the next best thing to actually speaking to people personally.

So we recorded our message, set up a special phone line that could handle multiple calls, and placed a small announcement in our local newspaper. At first there was just a trickle of calls. But as word of mouth spread, our phone line started to receive more and more calls. Within a short time we were getting dozens, then hundreds of calls a week. In a little more than five months our phone line had received more than six thousand calls. We were blown away by the response!

We even started to receive letters from people who were putting our simple guidelines into practice and getting positive results. This gave us a warm glow of pride.

But we did notice one thing. Many of the letters would finish by asking for even more information, particularly written information. It soon became obvious to us that although our phone line was certainly helpful, it simply wasn't enough. People needed more. And most important, they needed written information they could refer to.

So we worked hard in our spare time to achieve that goal, and for more than four years we compiled thousands of words about how to follow a MediterrAsian way of living.

We ended up condensing this information and presented it in a user-friendly format on the Internet in April 2004. We called our site MediterrAsian.com and, thanks again to positive word of mouth, it has now grown to become one of the most popular ethnic diet sites on the Internet. It has shown more than three million people how to incorporate traditional Mediterranean and Asian dietary and lifestyle practices into their own lives.

We see this book as an extension of our site, and we hope it gives you a good general understanding of the principles behind a MediterrAsian way of living. By following these principles, Trudy and I have profoundly changed our lives for the better. And we're confident that if you put these same simple principles into practice for yourself, your life will change for the better too.

Ric Watson, *January 2007*

Imagine for a moment that every day you could indulge in a large variety of tasty and satisfying foods such as pasta dishes, stir-fries, pizzas, curries, risottos, noodle dishes, and sushi, all washed down with a glass or two of your favorite wine or beer. Imagine as well that you never had to formally exercise and that you got to set aside special time every day to relax and unwind.

Now imagine that eating and living this way could help you: stay lean and healthy; substantially reduce your risk of contracting heart disease, diabetes, osteoporosis, and many types of cancer (including breast, prostate, and colon cancer); and increase your chances of living longer.

This way of living might sound like the impossible dream, but in reality people from Mediterranean and Asian cultures have been living like this, and reaping the rewards, for more than five thousand years.

TRADITIONAL DIETARY AND
LIFESTYLE PRACTICES

There's actually no such thing as a uniform Mediterranean or Asian diet and lifestyle. The Mediterranean region, for example, encompasses such diverse countries as Greece, Italy, Morocco, Turkey, Spain, and Tunisia. Not only do these countries share different ethnic, cultural, and religious backgrounds but the dishes traditionally eaten in these countries are also equally diverse and use a wide range of different cooking techniques as well as different herbs, spices, and seasonings.

The cultural and culinary diversity seen throughout the Mediterranean region is equally apparent in Asia, which includes such countries as Japan, China, Thailand, India, Vietnam, Indonesia, and Korea

Yet, despite the differences, research over the last fifty years has shown that there are also many distinct similarities between the traditional dietary and lifestyle practices of Mediterranean and Asian cultures:

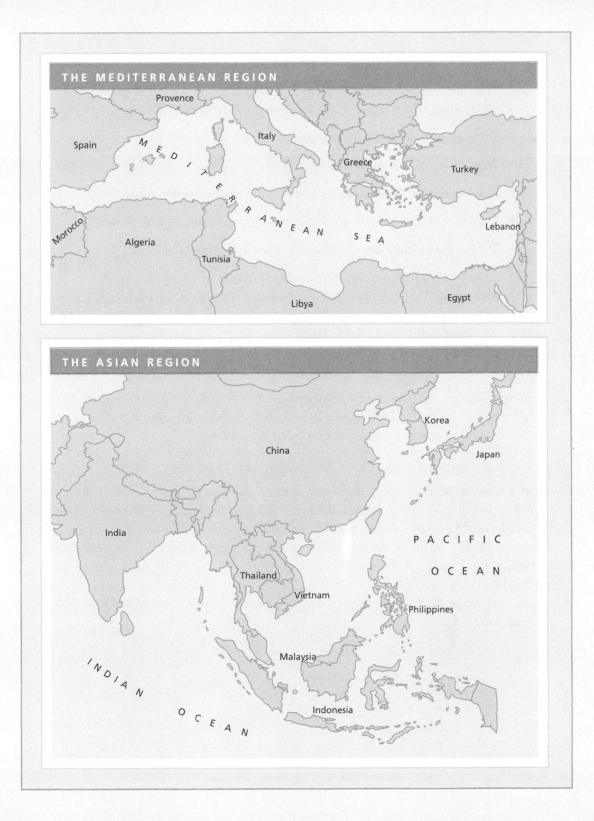

- Their diets include abundant amounts of plant foods such as grains, vegetables, fruits, legumes (beans, peas, and lentils), and nuts.

- They consume only small amounts of red meat.

- They consume fish regularly.

- Most of the fat they consume comes from plant and fish oils.

- They consume alcohol regularly in moderation (usually with meals).

- They are physically active as part of their everyday lives.

- They tend to have an optimistic view of life, family ties are strong, and special time is usually set aside each day to relax the body and mind (such as the afternoon siesta, common throughout the Mediterranean region, and Tai Chi and yoga, which are commonly practiced throughout Asia).

According to a large body of scientific research, these similar dietary and lifestyle practices help explain why Mediterranean and Asian peoples also share the same good health, low rates of chronic disease, and long life expectancy.

So how can a Westerner living in this fast-paced, high-stress modern world possibly adopt traditional Mediterranean and Asian dietary and lifestyle practices? If it sounds difficult, let us assure you that it's not. We both lead busy Western lives, and we've done it. In fact, for more than a decade we've been incorporating traditional Mediterranean and Asian dietary and lifestyle practices into our lives. Over that time, not only have we had lots of fun and discovered a world of wonderful tastes, but we've also experienced a remarkable improvement in our physical health and emotional well-being. And through this book, we'd like to show you how to easily follow a "MediterrAsian" way of living too.

Unlocking the Secrets of the Mediterranean Diet and the Asian Diet

One of the biggest benefits we've discovered in following a MediterrAsian way of living—along with how it makes us look and feel—is the peace of mind it gives us. With so many mixed messages out there, it's very comforting to know that a Medi-terrAsian lifestyle isn't based on unproven theories or current fads. It's based on what has worked for thousands of years.

And as well as being proven by the test of time, this lifestyle is also grounded in good science. In fact, for more than half a century, some of the Western world's top scientists and doctors have been endeavoring to unlock the secrets behind the exceptional health, lack of chronic disease, and long life enjoyed by the peoples of the Mediterranean region and Asia.

What they have discovered—and, in fact, are still discovering—is nothing short of remarkable.

THE GREAT CULTURAL DIVIDE

Scientists first started investigating the traditional dietary and lifestyle practices of Mediterranean and Asian cultures in the 1950s. They were looking for answers to why so many disorders common in Western society—such as coronary heart disease, breast cancer, diabetes, and obesity—were occurring frequently here, but very rarely there. What were these people doing that we weren't doing? Or was it simply a case of good genetics? The first person to attempt to answer that question was Ancel Keys, PhD, director of the Laboratory of Physiological Hygiene at the University of Minnesota School of Public Health.

Keys had already gained international notoriety in the 1940s for his research into the physiological effects of food and famine. Through his research he also developed a field survival ration for fighting troops, called the K Ration ("K" for Keys), which became the official combat ration for U.S. troops during World War II. By the 1950s, Keys's main focus was on preventing coronary heart disease, which was (and still is) the number one killer of both men and women in the Western world. He put forth a simple but powerful observation: "If some developed countries can do without heart attacks, why can't we?"

In the early 1950s, Keys traveled to the Mediterranean region, where, working closely with local physicians, he conducted a series of studies. The first study involved a group of firemen from Naples, in southern Italy. Keys found that the firemen were still eating the same Mediterranean-style diet that had sustained their ancestors for thousands of years: plenty of plant foods (including grains, beans, fruits, and vegetables); fish and seafood eaten regularly; very little animal foods; and olive oil as the primary source of fat. When blood tests were taken, Keys found that the firemen had significantly lower blood cholesterol levels than the Western average. But at this stage it was still unclear how much of a role genetics played.

Next Keys traveled to another part of the Mediterranean, Spain, where he conducted a study on two different groups of people living in Madrid. One group lived in the poor quarter of Madrid; the other group was made up of fifty professional Madrid businessmen. Keys found that the Madrid poor, like the firemen from Naples, were still eating a traditional Mediterranean-style diet. But he found that most of the Madrid businessmen had abandoned their traditional diet and were eating a diet comparable to that in the West, complete with large amounts of red meat and dairy foods and only small amounts of plant foods.

In both groups the genetics were the same, but Keys discovered that blood cholesterol levels varied significantly. The Madrid poor had low levels, whereas the Madrid businessmen had much higher levels and a correspondingly high rate of heart disease. Keys concluded that it was mainly the difference in diet that accounted for the greater incidence of heart disease among the businessmen.

To back up this observation, Keys turned his attention to Asia, which, like the Mediterranean, had rates of heart disease far lower than that generally found in Western society. In 1956 he set up a long-range study of Japanese people living in Japan, Hawaii, and Los Angeles. Keys found that Japanese living in Japan had significantly lower blood cholesterol levels and far lower rates of heart disease than Japanese who had migrated to Hawaii or Los Angeles and adopted a Western diet. And he made another intriguing finding: The traditional diet that seemed to be protecting the Japanese in Japan was very similar to the traditional diet he had seen in the Mediterranean—high in plant-based foods, moderate in fish, and low in animal foods.

Keys's studies produced the first firm evidence that diet played a major role in the onset of heart disease. Certain commercial interests—particularly the meat and dairy industries—still weren't convinced. But many others were, including the World Health Organization and President Eisenhower's heart specialist, Paul Dudley White. With their help, Keys began planning one of the largest and most comprehensive studies ever conducted into the link between diet and heart disease, the Seven Countries Study.

A GROUNDBREAKING STUDY

The Seven Countries Study was launched in 1958. For more than a decade, Professor Keys, with the help of an international team of specialists, studied the diet, lifestyle, and incidence of coronary heart disease among 12,763 randomly selected middle-aged men from seven countries: the United States, Japan, Italy, Greece, the Netherlands, Finland, and Yugoslavia.

When all the research was analyzed, a clear and predictable pattern emerged. In the Mediterranean and Asian regions of the world (specifically, Greece, Japan, and southern Italy)—where vegetables, grains, fruits, beans, and fish took center stage—heart disease was found to be rare. But in those countries where people filled their plates with red meat, cheese, and other foods high in saturated fat—such as in the United States and Finland—the rates of heart disease were found to be very high.

With hard figures from real populations, Keys was now certain that diet played the primary role in the onset of coronary heart disease. But, after so many years of research, he had come to realize that food might not be the only factor involved. Professor Keys

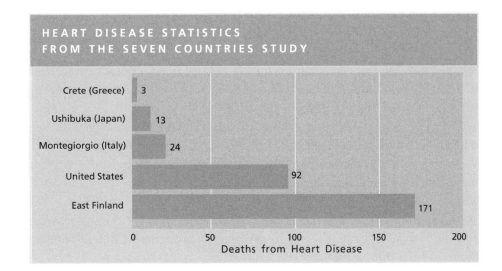

HEART DISEASE STATISTICS
FROM THE SEVEN COUNTRIES STUDY

Crete (Greece) 3
Ushibuka (Japan) 13
Montegiorgio (Italy) 24
United States 92
East Finland 171

Deaths from Heart Disease

also observed that Mediterranean and Asian peoples were physically active, family ties were strong, and the pace of life was leisurely. Keys concluded that although diet was the single most important factor, it was a combination of dietary and lifestyle factors that were responsible for the remarkably low rates of heart disease in Mediterranean and Asian regions.

The Seven Countries Study sparked a great deal of interest throughout the international scientific and medical communities. Dozens of studies on a molecular level followed in the 1970s and '80s, confirming Keys's findings. This led, in 1983, to the initiation of another large-scale population study. This time researchers concentrated their attention on Asia and in particular on China.

THE CHINA STUDY

The China-Cornell-Oxford Project (also known as the China Study) was conducted by Cornell University in the United States, Oxford University in England, and the Chinese Academy of Preventative Medicine. Launched in 1983, the massive study focused on China and involved dozens of researchers, led by T. Colin Campbell, PhD, professor of nutritional biochemistry at Cornell University. Between 1983 and 1990, researchers traveled across the far reaches of China—from the southern coastal regions to the Gobi desert—studying the dietary practices and disease rates among 10,200 Chinese men and women.

To make the study as comprehensive and thorough as possible, Dr. Campbell and his colleagues collected every conceivable piece of information they could about their subjects. They found that a rural Chinese diet was the same diet that had been eaten in China for thousands of years. It was rich in plant-based foods such as rice and vegetables, low in animal foods, and contained around three times more fiber than an average Western diet. The rates of heart disease and breast cancer in these areas were also found to be many times lower than in Western society, as were the rates for prostate cancer and osteoporosis. Obesity was also very rare.

But further research conducted on Chinese populations living outside rural areas told a different story. The research found that the diet in many urban areas of China was a lot more Westernized, with far more animal food consumption at the expense of traditional dietary staples like rice and vegetables. The study also revealed that the urban Chinese who had abandoned their traditional diet had much higher rates of common Western ailments than did their rural cousins, including heart disease, breast cancer, and prostate cancer. And obesity, which was rarely seen in rural Chinese populations, was found to be common among those Chinese eating a Westernized diet.

When the years of painstaking research were completed in 1990, the China Study had generated the largest database in the world on the multiple causes of disease. And the findings of the study were clear. "In the final analysis," reported Dr. Campbell, "we have strong evidence from this and other studies that nutrition becomes the controlling factor in the development of chronic degenerative diseases."

The China Study was hailed as a great success. Dr. Mark Hegsted, professor emeritus of nutrition at Harvard School of Public Health, called it "a very, very important study—unique and well done." The *New York Times* dubbed it the "Grand Prix of epidemiology" and went on to describe it as "the most comprehensive large study ever undertaken of the relationship between diet and the risk of developing disease . . . tantalizing findings."

The writing was now on the wall. It was clear that diet was the single most important factor in determining the onset of many chronic illnesses common in Western society. It was also clear that if people in the West wanted to live longer and reduce their risk of many chronic ailments, then the answer was to be found in adopting a traditional Mediterranean or Asian way of eating.

And two landmark studies have confirmed just how protective traditional Mediterranean and Asian diets can be for people who adopt them.

THE LYON DIET HEART STUDY

In 1988 Michel de Lorgeril, MD, from the University of Saint-Étienne in France, teamed up with researchers from the French National Center for Health Research to investigate the protective effects of a Mediterranean diet. In what became known as the Lyon Diet Heart Study, researchers randomly divided 605 male and female heart attack survivors into two groups. One group was advised to eat the standard, "prudent," low-fat diet suggested for heart patients. The other half were advised to eat a Mediterranean-style diet, complete with plenty of bread, pasta, olive oil, fresh vegetables, fruit, beans, small amounts of red meat, moderate amounts of fish and poultry, and wine with meals. Instead of butter, they were advised to use a canola oil–based spread.

Although the study was originally scheduled to last for five years, after only two years researchers were so astounded by the differences in the two groups that the study was abruptly ended for ethical reasons. It was found that those following the Mediterranean-style diet had a 70 percent lower death rate compared to those following the prudent low-fat diet. In a follow-up report, researchers also discovered that cancer rates among the Mediterranean group were 61 percent lower than those of the other group.

"The results were spectacular and of unexpected magnitude," reported Serge Renaud, PhD, from the French National Center for Health Research, Bordeaux, who helped initiate the study. "The protective effects of the diet began to occur within two months of observation."

In fact, the results of the Lyon Diet Heart Study—results that hadn't been seen in any other diet, drug, or medical trial—were deemed so important that they were published in three prestigious medical journals, the *American Journal of Clinical Nutrition*, the *Lancet*, and the *Journal of the American College of Cardiology*.

ASIAN-STYLE DIET ALSO SHOWS SIGNIFICANT BENEFITS

At the same time that French researchers were documenting the life-giving benefits of a Mediterranean-style diet, researchers in the United States were conducting a similar study into the role an Asian-style diet can play in reducing the risk of breast cancer in Western women.

In the study, conducted by a specialist team from the University of California, twenty-five breast cancer survivors were placed on an Asian-style diet and their progress was noted. Within only three months researchers saw biochemical changes in the breast in response to the change in diet.

John Glaspy, MD, director of the University of California Oncology Center and lead author of the study reported, "My colleagues and I have shown that at least one aspect of human breast composition in American women can be altered to approximate the breast composition of women in certain Asian and European countries . . . in those countries, the incidence of breast cancer is much lower than it is here." Researchers also noted that the Asian diet promoted better cardiovascular health as well as weight loss.

THE GREAT PYRAMIDS

With decades of research confirming the health-giving benefits of traditional Mediterranean and Asian dietary and lifestyle practices, members of the scientific and medical communities decided the time had come to fully educate the Western public on the merits of this way of living.

At an international conference in San Francisco, California, in 1994, a group of experts from three highly respected organizations—Harvard School of Public Health,

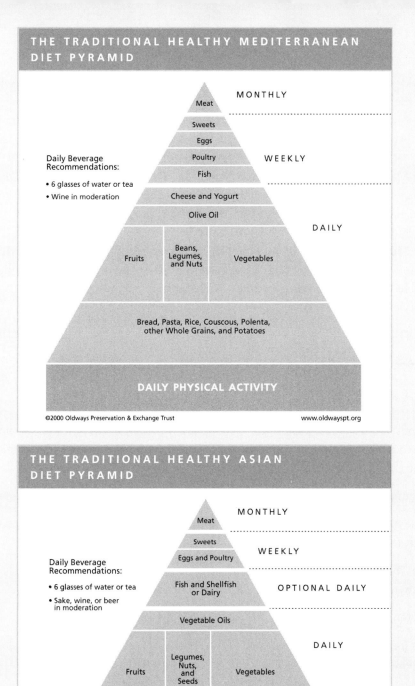

THE TRADITIONAL HEALTHY MEDITERRANEAN DIET PYRAMID

MONTHLY

Meat

Sweets

Eggs

Poultry — WEEKLY

Fish

Daily Beverage Recommendations:
- 6 glasses of water or tea
- Wine in moderation

Cheese and Yogurt

Olive Oil

DAILY

Fruits

Beans, Legumes, and Nuts

Vegetables

Bread, Pasta, Rice, Couscous, Polenta, other Whole Grains, and Potatoes

DAILY PHYSICAL ACTIVITY

©2000 Oldways Preservation & Exchange Trust   www.oldwayspt.org

THE TRADITIONAL HEALTHY ASIAN DIET PYRAMID

MONTHLY

Meat

Sweets

Eggs and Poultry — WEEKLY

Daily Beverage Recommendations:
- 6 glasses of water or tea
- Sake, wine, or beer in moderation

Fish and Shellfish or Dairy — OPTIONAL DAILY

Vegetable Oils

DAILY

Fruits

Legumes, Nuts, and Seeds

Vegetables

Rice, Noodles, Breads, Millet, Corn, and other Whole Grains

DAILY PHYSICAL ACTIVITY

©2000 Oldways Preservation & Exchange Trust   www.oldwayspt.org

the World Health Organization, and Oldways Preservation and Exchange Trust—released the *Traditional Healthy Mediterranean Diet Pyramid*.

The aim of the pyramid was simple: to illustrate, in a graphical form, the traditional healthy dietary and lifestyle practices of Mediterranean cultures. It was based on a culmination of research dating back to Professor Ancel Keys's first studies in the 1950s.

The Mediterranean Pyramid was followed in 1995 by the *Traditional Healthy Asian Diet Pyramid*, which was developed by the same organizations as the Mediterranean pyramid, and also by senior scientists from Cornell University, including Dr. T. Colin Campbell, director of the massive China Study.

The Mediterranean and Asian pyramids are marvelous blue prints of the traditional dietary and lifestyle characteristics of people from these areas. They also highlight the remarkable similarities between traditional Mediterranean and traditional Asian dietary and lifestyle practices.

TRADITIONAL DIETARY AND LIFESTYLE PRACTICES

MEDITERRANEAN	ASIAN
Grain foods such as bread, pasta, rice and couscous form a staple part of the daily diet.	Grain foods such as rice, noodles and millet form a staple part of the daily diet.
Fresh vegetables and fruits are eaten daily.	Fresh vegetables and fruits are eaten daily.
Vegetable oils and fish oils are the main sources of fat in the diet.	Vegetable oils and fish oils are the main sources of fat in the diet.
Red meat (beef, pork, and lamb) is eaten only a few times a month.	Red meat (beef, pork, and lamb) is eaten only a few times a month.
Fish is eaten regularly.	Fish is eaten regularly.
Legumes (beans, peas, and lentils) and nuts are eaten regularly.	Legumes (beans, peas, and lentils) and nuts are eaten regularly.
Alcohol, such as wine, is consumed daily in moderation.	Alcohol, such as beer and rice wine, is consumed daily in moderation.
Regular physical activity is an important part of everyday life.	Regular physical activity is an important part of everyday life.

Thanks to the publicity generated by the pyramids, many of us are now aware of the healthfulness of traditional Mediterranean and Asian dietary and lifestyle practices; the huge boom in sales of olive oil and soy products in recent years is testimony to that. But how do all the guidelines set out in the pyramids translate into real life for a Westerner living in this fast-paced modern world?

That's what the rest of this book is all about. Over the coming pages we'll go through these guidelines in detail. I'll outline why each one is so important and give you concrete, practical examples of how you can easily incorporate that guideline into your life. We'll also discuss one guideline that wasn't included in either the Mediterranean or Asian pyramid—the fact that Mediterranean and Asian cultures have known for centuries that emotional health is just as important as physical health. Indeed, more than two thousand years ago the Greek philosopher Aristotle defined the goal of all human endeavor as "happiness." We agree wholeheartedly!

Then we'll put all these guidelines together into a plan. Not just a plan for a month or a year, but a plan for *life*.

In the next chapter, we will start by looking at one of the most misunderstood nutrients in the Western world: fat.

Fat Fundamentals

Fat tastes great! It gives food a unique flavor and a feel in the mouth that's incomparable to any other type of food. And fat isn't only tasty, it's also an essential nutrient we need to survive.

Fat maintains cell membranes and blood vessels, it helps produce essential hormones that regulate numerous bodily functions, it provides your body with energy, and it helps maintain healthy skin and hair. Fat is also required in order to absorb the fat-soluble vitamins A, D, E, and K, which are essential for proper function of your eyes, immune system, and bones. But when it comes to fat, it's not all good news. The crucial fact is that not all fats are created equal.

SOME FATS HARM, SOME FATS HEAL

One of the biggest conclusions drawn from more than fifty years of research into eating patterns throughout the Mediterranean and Asia is that saturated fat (found in high amounts in red meat and dairy products) plays a pivotal role in the onset of many chronic diseases. At the same time, the weight of scientific evidence shows that unsaturated fat—found in high amounts in vegetable and fish oils—can actually help prevent disease.

Professor Ancel Keys saw firsthand how different types of fat can have vastly different effects on the chemistry of the body. During the 1950s Keys studied a group of woodchoppers in Finland, where heart disease rates were among the highest in the world.

Keys found that the diet of these men was very high in fat, particularly saturated fat from meat and dairy products. He even noted that many of the woodchoppers would butter their cheese. Keys found that a large percentage of these men were suffering from heart disease.

Later, during the Seven Countries Study, Keys conducted research on a group of villagers on the Greek island of Crete, where, along with Japan, heart disease rates were the lowest in the world.

Keys found that the Crete villagers, like the Finnish woodchoppers, also had a diet high in fat (up to 40 percent of their calories came from fat). But unlike the Finnish woodchoppers, who consumed lots of saturated fat from meat and dairy products, the fat in the Crete diets came primarily from olive oil and the oil in the fish they ate. Both of these oils are made up primarily of unsaturated fat. Keys found that these villagers had low blood-cholesterol levels, and heart disease amongst them was almost nonexistent.

So, what's the difference between saturated fat and unsaturated fat? And why do they behave so differently in the body? To really understand fat, it's important to learn a few basics first.

THE SKINNY ON FAT

Scientifically known as fatty acids, fats are divided into three main families: saturated fatty acids, polyunsaturated fatty acids, and monounsaturated fatty acids. The latter two are known collectively as unsaturated fats.

The major difference between these fatty acids lies in the type of molecules of which they're composed and the degree to which these molecules are saturated with hydrogen atoms.

Every type of fat, whether it's from a vegetable source or an animal source, actually contains a mixture of all three of these fatty acids. But, although all fats are made up of a mixture of saturated, polyunsaturated, and monounsaturated fatty acids, one type almost always predominates. And it's the fatty acid that predominates that classifies what type of fat it is.

For example, around 75 percent of the fatty acids in olive oil are monounsaturated, so scientists classify it as a monounsaturated fat. Safflower oil, on the other hand, contains around 75 percent of its fatty acids in the form of polyunsaturated fat, so it's known as a polyunsaturated fat. And animal fats, with between 50 and 70 percent of their fatty acids in the form of saturated fat, are classified as—you guessed it—saturated fat.

In general, fat from animal sources is high in saturated fat, and fat from vegetable sources is high in unsaturated fat. Tropical vegetable oils (palm oil and coconut oil) are the exception to this rule, and they contain an amount of saturated fatty acids similar to that found in animal fat.

THE DANGERS OF A DIET HIGH IN SATURATED FAT

One of the first clues that saturated fat is vastly different from unsaturated fat is the visible fact that highly saturated fat (such as butter and lard) is solid at room temperature, whereas highly unsaturated fat (such as olive and safflower oil) is liquid.

The chemical structure of saturated fat also affects how your body metabolizes it. Controlled clinical studies, as well as large population studies, have repeatedly shown that consuming too much saturated fat can lead to elevated levels of potentially harmful LDL cholesterol in the blood.

Our bodies are ill equipped to deal with large amounts of LDL cholesterol in the blood, and the excess can accumulate on the walls of our arteries. This can lead to the formation of plaque and to a hardening and narrowing of the arteries, known as *atherosclerosis*.

Atherosclerosis displays no symptoms as it gradually restricts blood flow. Eventually this can end up causing a clot (thrombus), completely blocking an artery that feeds blood to a vital organ. Ultimately this can lead to a heart attack if a coronary artery is

WHAT IS CHOLESTEROL?

Cholesterol (from the Greek words meaning "solid bile") is a soft, waxy substance that is found, to varying degrees, in everyone's body. We need cholesterol to survive, since it's used to form cell membranes and brain and nerve tissues. Cholesterol also helps the body produce hormones needed for body regulation, including processing food, and bile acids needed for digestion. Your liver actually produces all the cholesterol your body needs for these functions, so you don't need to consume any extra through your diet.

It used to be thought that eating dietary cholesterol was a major factor in raising potentially harmful LDL cholesterol levels in the blood; but in recent years studies have found that consuming dietary cholesterol has only a small effect. Consuming large amounts of bad fats (saturated and trans fats) has been identified as the main culprit.

Good and Bad Cholesterol

You may have heard about "bad" versus "good" cholesterol. Here's a simple explanation. Having high levels of LDL (low-density lipoprotein) cholesterol in your blood is considered bad because it can lead to a buildup of plaque inside your arteries, which can block the flow of blood to vital organs. HDL (high-density lipoprotein) cholesterol is considered good because it helps carry LDL cholesterol from the blood to the liver, where it can be naturally eliminated. An easy way to remember the difference is to think "H" for healthy and "L" for life-threatening.

Many of us are unaware of exactly how much fat red meat contains. The simple fact is that a large amount of the fat in red meat is hidden in tiny pockets within the flesh, so it's hard to gauge how much you are really eating. Here are some examples:

- An 8-ounce T-bone has more than 30 grams of fat.

- An 8-ounce burger patty has almost 35 grams of fat.

- An 8-ounce sirloin contains almost 40 grams.

This hidden fat isn't just bad for health; it can also affect how you look. Quite simply, hidden fat equals hidden calories, and red meat contains lots of calories. An 8-ounce sirloin steak, for example, contains more than 400 calories. This compares to an 8-ounce tuna steak, which contains only around 240 calories.

Researchers at the University of Michigan in Ann Arbor believe the high-calorie content of red meat could be one of the key reasons that many of us in the West are overweight. Several years ago they surveyed a group of obese men about what foods they liked the most; steaks and roasts topped the list.

But high cholesterol, atherosclerosis, and weight gain aren't the only problems caused by overconsumption of red meat. In recent years a number of major international studies have confirmed that eating large amounts of red meat can also increase your risk of contracting certain types of cancer, particularly breast, colon, and prostate cancer.

blocked, to stroke if an artery to the brain is blocked, or to kidney failure if an artery to the kidney is blocked.

Red Meat and Saturated Fat

The main source of saturated fat in a typical Western diet comes from red meat (beef, pork, and lamb). And red meat, in one form or another, usually takes center stage on most of our plates. Some typical examples include burgers, hot dogs, steak, meatloaf, bacon, spare ribs, roasts, meat pies, and sausages.

The opposite is true throughout Asia and the Mediterranean, where, for thousands of years, red meat has traditionally been reserved for special feast days, or eaten more as a garnish than a main course. Instead, the peoples of Asia and the Mediterranean have traditionally gotten their protein from highly unsaturated foods such as fish, shellfish, and plant foods, including beans and nuts.

This way of eating certainly makes sense because numerous studies have shown that red meat, and the high amounts of saturated fat it contains, elevates LDL-cholesterol levels and therefore raises the risk of arterial blockage.

THE CANCER CONNECTION

In late 1997 the World Cancer Research Fund and the American Institute for Cancer Research released the most comprehensive report of its kind into the link between diet and cancer. The report involved distinguished researchers from the United States, Britain, Japan, China, India, and Latin America, who reviewed more than 4,500 studies to come up with their detailed analysis, which was titled "Food, Nutrition and the Prevention of Cancer: A Global Perspective."

The report found that people who lived in areas like the Mediterranean and Asia, where red meat consumption is generally low and plant-food consumption is high, had the lowest rates of cancer in the world.

It was also found that when these healthy people moved to industrialized Western nations like the United States and Great Britain, where meat consumption is high and plant-food consumption low, their rate of cancers soon matched that of their adopted country. These population studies, plus strong evidence from thousands of clinical studies, led researchers to conclude that diet plays a vital role in preventing the onset of cancer.

The expert panel who prepared the report went on to recommend that if red meat is eaten at all, it should be limited to no more than 3 ounces per day, about the size of a deck of cards. Instead, it suggested eating fish and poultry.

Other large-scale studies have also shown a direct link between red meat consumption and increased risk of certain cancers. For example, Harvard scientists, who have been conducting an ongoing study involving more than 80,000 women since 1980, found that women who had beef, lamb, or pork as a daily main dish had two and a half times the risk of developing colon cancer as those who ate the meats less than once a month.

Prostate Cancer Linked to High Red-Meat Consumption

Prostate cancer is a leading cause of death for men in the Western world. Scientists have now identified red meat as a key risk factor. In one study, a group of researchers led by Dr. James Herbert of the University of Massachusetts Medical School reviewed a survey of prostate cancer deaths in fifty-nine countries. They found what a number of other studies have found: Prostate cancer deaths are much lower in countries where red meat is eaten rarely.

The researchers noted that the lowest death rates from prostate cancer are in countries such as Japan, where people traditionally eat a great deal of fish and very little red meat. "Animal energy was positively associated with prostate cancer mortality," commented Dr. Herbert. "On the other hand, intakes of cereals, soybeans, other nuts and oilseeds and fish were negatively associated with prostate cancer mortality."

The study concluded: "On the basis of the results of this study and other studies, it appears that the Western diet may contribute to the risk for prostate cancer mortality."

GRIM REPERCUSSIONS

As mentioned earlier, Asians and Mediterraneans have traditionally had very little red meat in their diets. Unfortunately, in recent years many Asians and Mediterraneans, particularly those living in urban areas, have started to abandon their traditional diets in favor of a Western diet high in red meat and low in plant foods. The results have been dramatic.

For example, since the 1970s, the Japanese diet has rapidly Westernized, and burgers, steaks, and processed foods have become increasingly popular, at the expense of the traditional Japanese staples of fish, vegetables, and rice. (Studies show that rice consumption in Japan has dropped by more than 50 percent in the last thirty years.) As this change in diet has occurred, there has also been a corresponding rise in obesity and the rates of heart disease and cancers of the colon, prostate, and breast. In fact, breast cancer, which used to be rare in Japan, rose by a dramatic 58 percent between 1975 and 1985, and it is still increasing at an alarming rate. Japanese researchers are convinced they know the reason why. In a *Time* magazine article, Dr. Akira Eboshida, chief deputy director of the Japanese Health and Welfare Ministry's Disease Control Division, said, "The largest factor behind the sharp rise is the Westernization of our eating habits. We are eating more animal fat and less fiber."

The traditional Mediterranean diet that has sustained Greeks for thousands of years has also started to Westernize since the 1970s, and the outcome has been identical to that seen in Japan. Professor Antonia Trichopoulou from the Greek National School of Public Health has been monitoring the changes. In the 1990s she published a study showing that a dramatic twenty-year rise in rates of heart disease and cancers of the breast and colon corresponded with a large increase in consumption of animal fats and a large decline in plant-food consumption.

The governments of Greece and Japan are now enthusiastically urging their citizens to return to the culinary traditions that have sustained their ancestors for thousands of years, the same culinary traditions presented in this book.

THE UNSATURATED FAT STORY

Monounsaturated and polyunsaturated fatty acids, which are collectively known as unsaturated fats, act in ways vastly different than saturated fat. For a start, instead of raising potentially dangerous LDL cholesterol in the blood, decades of research has shown they do just the opposite—they actually help lower it.

Unsaturated fats are also a rich source of vitamin E. This vitamin, as well as being an essential nutrient needed for a number of body-regulating functions, is also a powerful antioxidant, and antioxidants in their own right are thought to help prevent the buildup of cholesterol on artery walls. (See chapter 4, "Plant Power," for information about antioxidants.)

Polyunsaturated Fat

Polyunsaturated fat is actually divided into two groups: omega-6 polyunsaturated fatty acids (omega-6 fat) and omega-3 polyunsaturated fatty acids (omega-3s). Omega-6 fat is the primary fat in sunflower oil, corn oil, and safflower oil. It's also present in nuts and seeds, whole grains, and other plant foods. Omega-3s is found in fish and shellfish, particularly salmon, tuna, mackerel, sardines, and anchovies. It's also present in smaller amounts in dark green vegetables, walnuts, pecans, and flaxseeds.

You probably already know that vitamins are essential for good health, but did you know that polyunsaturated fats are just as essential? In fact, omega-3 and omega-6 fats are known scientifically as essential fatty acids, or EFAs. They're considered essential because they're not produced by the body, and they are necessary for a wide range of functions, including cell membrane formation, brain development, good eyesight, and the production of hormone-like compounds that regulate inflammation, blood pressure, heart rate, and immune response.

Monounsaturated Fat

Although monounsaturated and polyunsaturated fats both lower your blood cholesterol levels, monounsaturated fat has been shown to do this more effectively. Omega-6 polyunsaturated fat lowers potentially harmful LDL cholesterol, but it tends to also slightly lower good HDL cholesterol. Studies have shown that monounsaturated fat, on the other hand, lowers LDL without affecting heart-protective HDL levels. In one study, researchers from Pennsylvania State University and the University of Rochester in New York found that when twenty-two subjects consumed a diet rich in monounsaturated fat from olive oil, peanuts, and peanut oil, their LDL cholesterol levels dropped by an average of 14 percent in four weeks. At the same time, there was no change in heart-protective HDL cholesterol levels. "These results show that eating more monounsaturated fat can reduce your heart-disease risk by 25 percent," reported Penny

Kris-Etherton, the study author and a professor in the Pennsylvania State University's Department of Nutrition.

Recent research has also shown that monounsaturated fat has many other health-giving benefits. A study published in the *Archives of Internal Medicine*, for example, shows that olive oil can lower blood pressure and make blood pressure–lowering medications less necessary.

The study involved twenty-three people on medication to control high blood pressure, who were divided into two groups. Both groups ate a nutritionally balanced diet that was identical, except for the type of oil used.

During the first six months of the study, one group used olive oil (a highly monounsaturated fat), while the other group used sunflower oil (which is made up primarily of omega-6 polyunsaturated fat). During the last six months of the study, the two groups switched the type of oil they used. It was found that when the participants used olive oil, their systolic (top number) and diastolic (bottom number) blood pressure fell by an average of seven points; but sunflower oil had no effect. As blood pressure decreased, researchers adjusted the participants' medication regimen. Olive oil was so effective at reducing blood pressure that many patients reduced their drug dosage by half, and eight went off blood-pressure drugs entirely.

Another study suggests that monounsaturated fat can also help maintain brainpower into old age. This time researchers from the University of Bari in Italy, led by Dr. Antonio Capurso, studied a group of 278 senior citizens. Those who consumed diets high in monounsaturated fat were found to be less likely to experience age-related cognitive decline compared with people who ate less monounsaturated fat.

Dr. Capurso concluded: "It appears that high monounsaturated fatty acid intakes, mostly present in vegetable oils and particularly in extra-virgin olive oil, the main fat of the Mediterranean diet, protect from age-related cognitive decline."

The Weight-Loss Bonus

Monounsaturated fat may even help you lose weight and maintain that loss, according to a study by researchers at Brigham and Women's Hospital and Harvard Medical School.

In the study sixty-one overweight men and women consumed one of two diets: a standard low-fat diet or a Mediterranean-style diet with regular moderate consumption of healthy monounsaturated fat from olive oil, olives, nuts, and nut products (such as nut oils and peanut butter). Both groups were instructed to consume the same number of calories.

After six months both groups had experienced roughly the same amount of weight loss, but the big difference came at the end of the study, twelve months later. It was found that a large number of the Mediterranean diet group had stuck with the diet and maintained their weight loss. However, many of those on the low-fat diet couldn't stick with it and had not only regained their lost weight, but weighed more than they did before the study began. "In our study, three times as many people trying to lose weight were able to stick to a Mediterranean-style diet versus the low-fat diet," reported the lead author of the study, Kathy McManus, RD, director of nutrition at Brigham and Women's Hospital. She noted that "patients loved this diet because they could include favorite foods if they carefully watched portion sizes."

The researchers concluded: "Motivation and adherence are very hard to sustain in any weight loss programs, but the results from this study suggest that the tastier the food, the greater overall success of the diet plan—even if it does include moderate amounts of fat."

NEW FAT ON THE BLOCK

We've looked at the different roles of saturated, polyunsaturated, and monounsaturated fat, but there's also a "synthetic" fat that's important to mention.

Early in the twentieth century scientists discovered they could create a new kind of fat by injecting hydrogen molecules into vegetable oil. This made the oil, which was normally liquid at room temperature, into a solid type of fat. The more hydrogen added to the oil, the harder the resulting fat. This process, called hydrogenation, is used to turn vegetable oil into margarine and vegetable shortening.

Although hydrogenated fats have some advantages over normal vegetable oils—namely, they have a longer shelf life and can be heated to higher temperatures—studies have shown that these fats can be even more dangerous to your health as saturated fat.

The trouble lies in the fact that when liquid oils are turned solid through the process of hydrogenation, this changes the building blocks of the fat and creates what are called trans fatty acids, or trans fats for short. Research has shown that trans fat raises bad cholesterol levels, lowers good cholesterol, and raises triglycerides (blood fats)—all of which are known risk factors for heart disease.

A typical Western diet is very high in trans fats because margarine has become increasingly popular and hydrogenated vegetable fats are used in everything from cookies, crackers, and pastries to fried snack foods like potato chips and foods fried in fast-food outlets.

"It's fat that makes you fat," proclaim the low-fat diet gurus. "No, you're quite wrong," say the low-carbohydrate gurus, "carbohydrates make you fat." Meanwhile, we're stuck in the middle, trying to figure out who's right.

Well, the truth is, they're both partly right. Yes, fat can make you fat; but so can carbohydrates—and, in fact, so can protein. Here's how it works.

All foods are made up of macronutrients. The three macronutrients are fat, protein, and carbohydrates. All three macronutrients contain stored energy, which scientists call kilocalories, or calories for short. (Vitamins and minerals, which are called micronutrients, contain no calories.) The three macronutrients are used in various ways by the body.

1. Protein is used primarily for building, repairing, and maintaining muscles, making blood cells, and synthesizing hormones and enzymes.

2. Carbohydrates are broken down into glucose (blood sugar) in the body. Glucose fuels your muscles and gives them energy to work; it's also the primary fuel for the brain and the central nervous system.

3. Fat is used for energy and is also an essential building block for the body's cells and is required in order to absorb fat-soluble vitamins.

If you eat more macronutrients than your body needs for these purposes and you don't burn them off through physical activity, those excess calories are converted into fat and stored on your body.

"Whether you store fat or don't store fat has to do with caloric balance," explains Alice Lichtenstein, DSc, a scientist at the Jean Mayer USDA Human Nutrition Research Center on Aging at Tufts University in Boston. "If you eat too many extra calories as protein, you'll store them as body fat, just as you would too many calories from carbohydrate."

Proof that calories are the only thing that matters in weight control was shown in a 1996 study where two groups of obese people were fed diets equally low in calories but different in their fat and carbohydrate content. One group received a diet with 15 percent carbohydrates and 53 percent fat; the other group got 45 percent carbohydrates and 26 percent fat. The researchers found there was no difference in weight loss between the two groups, and they concluded that it was the number of calories eaten, not the proportion of calories from carbohydrates or fat, that determined weight loss.

continues on next page

Calories Count, but Don't Count Calories

So, when it comes to maintaining a healthy weight, it's calories that count. But that certainly doesn't mean you have to count calories to stay in shape. Remember, for thousands of years Mediterraneans and Asians have kept lean and trim, yet they had absolutely no idea what a calorie was (this is a modern scientific term). They simply ate food that tasted good and made them feel good.

Coincidentally the majority of this food also happens to be bulky, filling, and satisfying but only moderate in calories. The great benefit of this way of eating is that it means you'll feel full and satisfied long before the calories can do any damage. Later in the book we'll show you just how easily this principle works in real life (see page 94).

OIL CHANGE:

HOW TO EAT LESS BAD FAT AND MORE GOOD FAT

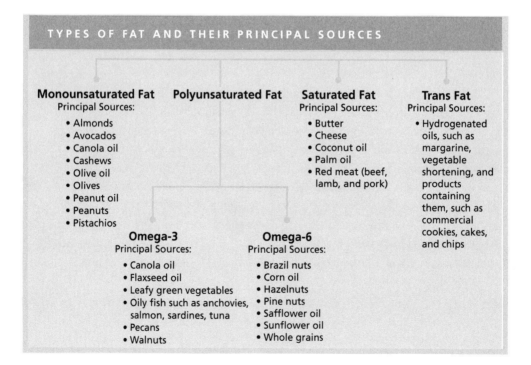

TYPES OF FAT AND THEIR PRINCIPAL SOURCES

Monounsaturated Fat
Principal Sources:
- Almonds
- Avocados
- Canola oil
- Cashews
- Olive oil
- Olives
- Peanut oil
- Peanuts
- Pistachios

Polyunsaturated Fat

Omega-3
Principal Sources:
- Canola oil
- Flaxseed oil
- Leafy green vegetables
- Oily fish such as anchovies, salmon, sardines, tuna
- Pecans
- Walnuts

Omega-6
Principal Sources:
- Brazil nuts
- Corn oil
- Hazelnuts
- Pine nuts
- Safflower oil
- Sunflower oil
- Whole grains

Saturated Fat
Principal Sources:
- Butter
- Cheese
- Coconut oil
- Palm oil
- Red meat (beef, lamb, and pork)

Trans Fat
Principal Sources:
- Hydrogenated oils, such as margarine, vegetable shortening, and products containing them, such as commercial cookies, cakes, and chips

Following are the five most effective ways of replacing bad fats in your diet with good fats.

First, instead of making red meat the main source of protein in your diet, opt for fish, shellfish, poultry, legumes, and nuts. Because red meat is the main source of saturated fat in a typical Western diet, the ideal first step in any plan to lower saturated fat intake is to reduce your intake of red meat. But at the same time it's important to remember that red meat only becomes a health hazard when you eat too much of it. Learning from the traditions of Asia and the Mediterranean region, it would seem that the key word is *moderation* not *elimination*.

A steak, some bacon, or a hamburger once in a while won't do you any harm. It's only when you start eating too much of these types of food—which is easy to do in our "meat-loving" culture—that the problems can start arising.

Of course, the thought of cutting back on red meat usually leads to the inevitable question: "Where am I going to get my protein?" Our answer: from *fish, shellfish, poultry, legumes (beans, peas,* and *lentils), nuts, and seeds.* This is where Mediterranean and Asian cultures have gotten their protein from for the last few thousand years. Like red meat, these foods are packed with protein, but unlike red meat, which is typically loaded with saturated fat, these foods contain mostly heart-healthy unsaturated fats.

But all this doesn't mean much if these foods don't taste good. The great news is that over the centuries the humble home cooks of Asia and the Mediterranean have discovered a myriad of ways to turn fish, shellfish, poultry, beans, and nuts into delicious, sometimes extraordinary dishes. The recipe section of this book will give you a good idea of what I mean.

Second, make olive, peanut, and canola (rapeseed) oils your main cooking fats. These are traditionally the main cooking oils used throughout the Mediterranean and Asia. All these oils are also made up primarily of monounsaturated fat, which lowers LDL cholesterol without affecting good HDL cholesterol. This makes them the obvious first choice as your main cooking oil.

Let's look at these oils in a bit more detail:

Olive oil. Throughout the Mediterranean region, olive oil has been revered as one of the basic staffs of life for thousands of years. There are three main varieties of olive oil: extra-virgin, virgin, and pure.

Extra-virgin olive oil—made from the first "cold pressing" (which means the oil is extracted with pressure, and no chemicals are involved) of the highest-quality olives—has a greenish tinge and a wonderfully rich aromatic taste. It also has very low acidity levels, generally no more than 1 percent. This low acidity means that extra-virgin olive oil lasts longer than other varieties of olive oil, but it also gives it a low smoking point, making it unsuitable for cooking at very high temperatures (although it's fine for lightly frying and sautéing). Another good use for extra-virgin olive oil is to add it to food near the end of the cooking process as a texture and flavor enhancer. It goes particularly well with pasta dishes, grilled fish or vegetables, and stews; in salad dressings, marinades, sauces, and soups; or simply drizzled over a piece of fresh crusty bread.

Virgin olive oil is produced in the same way as extra-virgin oil, but it uses lower-grade olives. This gives it a less pronounced flavor and higher acidity levels (around 3 percent) than extra-virgin oil, which means that its smoking point is higher.

Pure olive oil (which is available in standard and extra-light varieties) is made by extracting oil from the leftover pulp from the process of making virgin and extra-virgin olive oils. This is done using heat and chemical extraction methods instead of cold pressing. Pure olive oil is cheaper and has a milder taste than the other two varieties of olive oil. It also has a higher smoking point, making it suitable for most cooking purposes, including barbecuing and frying.

From a health point of view, extra-virgin and virgin olive oils are the best choices because the oil has been removed without heat, which means the heat-sensitive vitamins and antioxidants are preserved.

Canola oil (rapeseed oil).

Rapeseed oil has been used in Asian cooking for centuries. Most of us know rapeseed oil by its other name, canola oil. Actually canola is a type of rapeseed oil that was developed by Canadian scientists in the 1970s and is milder and more easily digested than normal rapeseed oil.

It's one of the most versatile oils because it has very little flavor and a high smoking point. We use it at home as our all-purpose cooking oil, and it's perfect for stir-fries, curries, and baked dishes.

In the health stakes, canola oil is also a winner. Not only is it made up mostly of heart-healthy monounsaturated fats but around 10 percent of its fat content is in the form of omega-3 fatty acids, which are essential for good health.

Peanut oil. This is another oil that has been traditionally used in Asian cooking for generations. Like canola oil, it's mild in flavor and has a high smoking point, so it's good for general-purpose use (it's a particularly good stir-fry oil). We often alternate between peanut oil and canola oil in our cooking.

Third, eat less trans fat–packed snacks and more nuts. Snacks like potato chips, cookies, and pastries typically contain lots of trans fats. On the other hand, nuts (such as walnuts, cashews, almonds, and pistachios) contain healthy unsaturated fats as well as vitamins, minerals, and dietary fiber. Just keep in mind that nuts contain a fair number of calories. Depending on the type of nut, an ounce, which is about a handful, has between 165 and 200 calories. So the idea is to enjoy nuts regularly but in moderation and particularly as a substitute for less wholesome snacks.

Fourth, instead of spreading bread with butter or margarine, use avocado, hummus, natural peanut butter, or trans fat–free margarine. When studies started showing the dangers of a diet high in saturated fat, many of us switched from butter to margarine to save our arteries from becoming clogged. But now scientists are telling us margarine isn't such a healthy alternative after all because of the potentially dangerous trans fat it contains. (It can really start to seem like a case of damned if you do, damned if you don't!)

So what's the best solution? We believe it comes down to being a bit creative and finding ways of substituting bad fats for good fats. For example, instead of using butter or margarine on your sandwich, try mashed avocado instead. The fat in avocados is mostly monounsaturated, so you get all the creaminess of butter or margarine without the guilt. Hummus (a Middle Eastern chickpea and sesame seed dip and spread) is another good alternative because it's also creamy, but it contains mostly unsaturated fat.

You could also use peanut butter as the spread, because the fat in peanuts is mostly monounsaturated. But a word of warning: Use *natural* peanut butter with no added vegetable oil. The vegetable oil in most commercial peanut butters is hydrogenated vegetable oil, which is high in trans fat.

If you're having bread or rolls at the side of your meal, instead of serving it with butter or margarine, do what Mediterraneans traditionally do—serve it with a small dish of extra-virgin olive oil for dipping or drizzling. You can also use olive oil instead of butter or margarine to make garlic bread.

If you've still got a hankering for something that tastes like and resembles butter, you're in luck. In response to the highly publicized side effects caused by trans fat, many manufacturers now offer trans fat–free margarine in tubs. These are a great alternative to butter or normal margarine; especially if you select a brand that uses a monounsaturated fat like canola or olive oil as its base.

Fifth, consume dairy products in moderation. After red meat, the second largest source of saturated fat in a typical Western diet comes from dairy foods (milk, cheese, butter, cream, and yogurt).

Throughout most of Asia (except the Indian subcontinent), dairy foods have traditionally played almost no role in the diet. A traditional Mediterranean diet, on the other hand, does include a moderate amount of dairy. But, unlike in Western society, Mediterraneans traditionally have consumed very little butter or milk (these foods quickly spoiled in the hot Mediterranean climate). Most of their dairy intake has been in the form of cheese or yogurt. Even then, this type of food has been seen as an accompaniment to meals, and was mostly used in small amounts to add texture and flavor to dishes. The cheese was often a strong cheese like Parmesan, which also meant a little went a long way.

Of course, one of the biggest concerns in the West about cutting down on dairy food intake is the belief that it will inevitably lead to osteoporosis, the bone thinning disease. I remember constantly being told as a kid, "If you don't drink your milk, you won't grow up with strong teeth and bones." But science is now discovering that's not quite the case.

There is no doubt that calcium is good for your bones, and there is no doubt that dairy products are a good source of calcium. The trouble is that dairy products aren't the ideal food source for delivering calcium to your body, because they are also high in animal protein. For more than thirty years studies have shown that if we consume too much animal protein, it tends to leech calcium from our bones. So by consuming lots of dairy products, we are naturally also consuming lots of animal protein and leeching out calcium almost as fast as we're receiving it.

A Harvard study involving more than 80,000 women found that increased calcium consumption through milk did not decrease osteoporosis risk at all. In fact, those who drank three glasses of milk a day had more hip and wrist fractures (a common measure of the extent of osteoporosis) than those who rarely drank milk. A similar study in Australia showed identical results.

And the facts speak for themselves. In countries where dairy consumption is high—such as in the United States, Britain, and Australia—osteoporosis rates are also high. But in parts of the world where dairy product consumption is much lower, such as in Asia and the Mediterranean, osteoporosis rates are also low.

In the massive China Study, for example, researchers from Cornell University found that rural Chinese people rarely consumed dairy products, yet their rates of osteoporosis were among the lowest in the world.

Dr. T. Colin Campbell, who led the study, points out, "Dairy calcium is not needed to prevent osteoporosis. Most Chinese consume no dairy products and, instead, get all their calcium from vegetables."

And this is by far the best way to get your calcium. Sure, you can still get some calcium through dairy foods. The trick is to eat dairy foods in moderation, as the Mediterraneans traditionally have. This ensures that your animal protein intake won't go overboard, and calcium won't be leeched out of your bones. At the same time, it also means you'll automatically be cutting down on saturated fat.

The best calcium-rich plant foods are dark green vegetables, beans (including tofu), nuts, and fruit. And as a bonus, fresh produce like this also contains high levels of magnesium and potassium, which are other important minerals that are needed for strong, healthy bones.

This chapter has explored the subject of fat in lots of detail. I hope you now have a good basic understanding of the different types of fats, and the vastly different effects they have on your body.

But there is one type of fat that I have touched on only briefly in this chapter: omega-3 fatty acids. This special fat has been the focus of a great deal of research in recent years, and because the richest source of omega-3 is fish and shellfish, I've saved most of the details about this extraordinary fat for the next chapter, which deals exclusively with seafood. And the great news—as you're about to find out—is that fish and shellfish aren't only a delicious source of healthy omega-3s, they also have many other remarkable health-giving benefits.

A Feast of Health from the Sea

For the past few thousand years the abundant waters of the Mediterranean Sea, Pacific Ocean, and Indian Ocean have provided the peoples of the Mediterranean region and Asia with a treasure trove of edible delights. Some of the mouthwatering seafood plucked from these waters includes shrimp, salmon, crab, tuna, lobster, mussels, squid, oysters, and scallops.

And none of these delightful morsels go to waste either, because fish and shellfish are as popular throughout Asia and the Mediterranean region as red meat is in the West. In Japan, for example, people consume an average of more than 80 pounds of fish and seafood per person each a year (this compares to only 15 pounds per person each year in the United States).

Researchers now believe this high consumption of fish and shellfish could partly help to explain why people in Mediterranean and Asian countries live longer, are leaner, and suffer from far less heart disease than we do.

So, what is the secret ingredient that makes fish and shellfish so healthy? Well, there are actually several reasons why these are among the most life-giving foods known to science, but a good place to start would be with the special fat found in fish and shellfish called *omega-3 fatty acids*, or omega-3s for short.

As you found out in the last chapter, this special fat, along with omega-6, is an essential fat we need to consume regularly to stay healthy. Research in recent years has also shown that omega-3s not only promote good health but can also help prevent a wide range of illnesses common in Western society. An area of particular interest has been the ability of omega-3 to lower the risk of heart disease.

OMEGA-3 FATTY ACID CONTENT IN FISH AND SHELLFISH		
VERY GOOD SOURCE	GOOD SOURCE	MODERATE SOURCE
Anchovy	Cod, Pacific	Catfish
Herring	Flounder	Clams
Mackerel	Halibut	Cod, Atlantic
Salmon	Oysters	Crab
Sardines	Perch, ocean	Crayfish
Swordfish	Pollock	Fish sticks (whitefish)
Trout	Rockfish	Haddock
	Scallops	Lobster
	Tuna, fresh	Shrimp
	Tuna, white, canned	Snapper
	Whiting	Tuna, light, canned

OMEGA-3 AND HEART DISEASE

For hundreds of years it has been known that people who consume fish regularly show striking patterns of good health. But it wasn't until research in the 1960s and '70s that omega-3 fatty acids were first isolated as being one of the primary health-giving components of fish. Studies during that time showed that Japanese fishermen and Greenland Eskimos, who consumed fish regularly, had very low rates of heart disease. Tests revealed that both the Japanese fishermen and the Greenland Eskimos also had high amounts of omega-3s in their blood. Further research found that omega-3s helped thin the blood and inhibit the onset of atherosclerosis (clogged arteries). Researchers concluded that regularly eating fish rich in omega-3s could help reduce the risk of heart disease.

This research was widely publicized in the media and is now familiar to many of us. But the research on omega-3s certainly didn't stop there. Dozens of clinical trials and population studies have now been conducted showing that not only the Japanese and Greenland Eskimos but Mediterraneans, Dutch, and Americans who eat fish frequently also have less risk of heart disease.

In one study—involving 827 people matched for age, sex, weight, and family history of heart disease—researchers at the University of Washington, Seattle, found that the intake of just one portion of fatty fish a week (fatty fish is the best source of omega-3) equaled a 50 percent lower risk of heart attack.

How Omega-3 Helps Prevent Heart Disease

Scientists believe there are several reasons omega-3s are so heart healthy. First, omega-3 has been shown to significantly reduce blood-platelet cell stickiness (platelets are one of the components in blood that causes clotting). Research has also shown that omega-3 can slow down the buildup of cholesterol in the arteries, which makes heart disease less likely.

It appears that omega-3 can even change the chemistry in the heart affecting heartbeat, the flow of blood, and chemical reactions in the blood vessels. "Potentially what happens is that fish actually can quiet the heart cells that might be irritated in a heart attack or during a period where the heart is not getting enough blood supply due to blockages in the arteries," says Dr. Christine Albert, who was involved in an eleven-year Harvard University study involving more than 21,000 people, which showed that just one serving of omega-3 rich fish weekly equaled a 52 percent reduction in sudden heart attack death.

On top of this, omega-3 has also been shown to help reduce blood-pressure and high triglyceride (blood-fat) levels, both of which are known risk factors for heart disease.

When you combine all these elements together, it's easy to see why omega-3s are one of the most powerful natural defenses against heart disease known to science.

Omega-3 and Stroke

Since omega-3s help prevent the arteries of the heart from becoming blocked, not surprisingly the rate of thrombotic stroke (stroke caused by a blockage to the arteries leading to the brain) has also been found to be much lower among those people who eat fish regularly.

In a study involving more than 80,000 women, researchers from Harvard School of Public Health found that women who ate five or more servings of fish a week had one-third the risk of a thrombotic stroke compared to women who ate fish once a month or less.

"I wasn't surprised by the direction of this study, but I was surprised by the magnitude," reported Dr. Meir Stampfer, professor of nutrition and epidemiology at the Harvard School of Public Health and a coauthor of the study. "I didn't expect the protective effect of fish to be that strong."

BRAIN FOOD

Remember how your grandmother told you fish was good brain food? Well, these classic words of wisdom are now being backed up by modern science.

The brain is actually made up of more than 50 percent fat, and research has found that the most abundant of these fats is a type of omega-3 fatty acid called DHA (docosahexaenoic acid). Studies have shown that DHA is a crucial building block of the brain that enhances brain-cell communication and nerve-signal transmission. Other research has shown that diets that don't contain enough DHA-rich omega-3s can lead to behavioral changes, learning difficulties, and a change in the biochemistry of the brain. This means that omega-3s have wide-ranging effects on the healthy functioning of your brain, including your susceptibility to depression.

OMEGA-3 AND DEPRESSION

Researchers have found an interesting relationship between consumption of omega-3s and the incidence of depression. In countries where fish consumption is low, depression rates tend to be high. On the other hand, in countries where fish consumption is high, depression rates tend to be low. Studies have also found that people with depression often have low levels of omega-3 in their cells, and these people typically respond well to an increase in omega-3 in their diet.

Groundbreaking research is now showing that increasing the consumption of omega-3s can even have positive results in treating the most severe form of depression, bipolar disorder (manic depression). In one study by researchers at Harvard Medical School, a group of thirty people diagnosed with bipolar disorder were divided into two groups. One group received supplements of omega-3-rich fish oil while the other group was given a placebo.

After four months researchers found that the group receiving fish oil had a significantly longer period of remission from illness than the placebo group. The patients who received the fish oil also displayed considerable improvement on tests assessing levels of depression and other bipolar symptoms.

Dr. Andrew L. Stoll, who led the study, believes there are several reasons why omega-3 rich fish oil was so effective at reducing depression. "Fish oil blocked the abnormal signaling in the brain which we think is present in mania and depression," he reported. He also noted that fish oil boosted levels of the neurotransmitter serotonin in the brain, similar to the effect of popular antidepressant drugs such as Prozac.

OMEGA-3 AND ALZHEIMER'S DISEASE

Because of the ability of omega-3s to improve brain function, it's not surprising that this remarkable fat has also been shown to be of benefit in reducing the risk of developing Alzheimer's disease. In a study of more than 1,000 people (average age seventy-five), those with high blood levels of omega-3 were found to be more than 40 percent less likely to develop Alzheimer's over a period of nine years than people with low omega-3 levels. Research by Danish scientists who compared the diets of 5,386 healthy older men and woman also found that the more fish in a person's diet, the lower his or her risk of developing Alzheimer's disease.

OMEGA-3 AND ARTHRITIS

New research is constantly finding ways in which omega-3s can be beneficial to our health. Another area where omega-3 has shown great potential is with inflammatory illnesses such as arthritis and asthma.

In one study, by Dr. Jean A. Shapiro in association with the Fred Hutchinson Cancer Research Institute, Seattle, Washington, researchers used a food frequency questionnaire to compare 324 rheumatoid arthritis cases with 1,245 controls. They found that those who ate an average of just two servings a week of omega-3 rich fish were 57 percent less likely to develop rheumatoid arthritis as those who ate less than one.

Nearly two dozen studies have also shown that people with rheumatoid arthritis have less fatigue and joint stiffness and could lower their anti-inflammatory drugs when they increased their intake of omega-3.

FISH: THE WEIGHT-LOSS SUPERFOOD

Fish is moderate in calories, yet filling and satisfying. In effect, this means that if you eat more fish, particularly in place of high-calorie red meat, losing weight should happen naturally. It certainly did for champion Australian weight lifter Dean Lukin.

Dean won the gold medal for weight lifting in the superheavyweight division at the 1984 Los Angeles Olympics. And Dean was certainly a superheavyweight himself, tipping the scales at over 300 pounds. But after his weight-lifting career ended, Dean was desperate to lose the pounds—not just to look better but to generally improve his health.

Dean decided to cut back on the highly processed foods and red meat that had made him fat. Instead, he adopted a diet resembling that of previous generations of his family, who came from the Mediterranean region and ate a diet that included fish as their main source of protein. "My father grew up in a seaside village on the Dalmatian coast (part of the Mediterranean region) and he and his family basically lived off the sea," recalls Dean in his 1993 book, *The Dean Lukin Diet*. "My great-grandfather lived until he was ninety-six. My grandfather's brother is still going strong in his 90s, so I figure the stuff can't be all that bad for you!"

Dean came to the conclusion that a weight-loss program using fish as the main source of protein would be the commonsense way to go. And he soon discovered there was a big bonus to eating a diet that included lots of moderate-calorie fish: "I found that I can eat larger quantities of fish than most other foods without putting on weight—being a person who's big on volume I find it ideal."

So, what happened when Dean started eating like his Mediterranean relatives? He ended up losing an incredible 110 pounds of fat in less than a year, or as Dean puts it: "When I got to the stage of really ripping the blubber off, the rate of progress was quite startling." Just as incredible is the fact that, as I write, he has kept that weight off for well over a decade.

Of course, Dean doesn't put all his success down to eating more fish. He followed his Mediterranean relatives and also increased his consumption of highly nutritious vegetables, fruits, and grain-based foods such as pasta and rice. He also made sure he kept active. But Dean reckons that eating plenty of fish was a major contributing factor to his dramatic weight loss.

HIGH IN "QUALITY" PROTEIN

In the West we often base our meals around red meat such as beef, pork, or lamb. These foods all contain plenty of protein, which your body needs for growth and repair. Unfortunately, they also contain large amounts of saturated fat, which your body most certainly doesn't need.

Fish and shellfish, on the other hand, contain just as much protein as red meat, but instead of containing lots of bad fat they contain good fat. The protein found in all seafood is also identical to that found in red meat, and is a "complete" protein. This means it contains all the essential amino acids (the building blocks of protein) your body needs for repair and growth.

VITAMIN AND MINERAL RICH

A s well as being a rich source of protein, fish and shellfish also contain high amounts of many important vitamins and minerals that are essential for optimal health.

VITAMIN AND MINERAL CONTENT OF FISH AND SHELLFISH		
NUTRIENT	BEST FISH AND SHELLFISH SOURCES	MAIN ROLE
Vitamin A	Crab, halibut, salmon, sardines, swordfish, tuna, whitefish	Maintains healthy skin, bones, teeth, and vision
Vitamin B12	Crab, herring, mackerel, oysters, salmon, trout	Needed for making red blood cells and maintaining the central nervous system
Vitamin E	Anchovies, haddock, herring, mackerel, salmon, sardines, tuna	An important antioxidant that protects body cells from free-radical damage
Vitamin D	Anchovies, mackerel, salmon, sardines, tuna	Promotes strong bones and teeth and helps with the absorption of calcium and phosphorus
Calcium	Herring, oysters, salmon, sardines, shrimp	Builds bones and teeth, regulates blood clotting, and is essential for normal functioning of nerves and muscles
Iron	Anchovies, abalone, clams, mackerel, mussels, oysters, perch, salmon, sardines, shrimp, trout, tuna	Needed for making red blood cells and transporting oxygen in blood and muscles
Phosphorus	Cod, halibut, perch, salmon, scallops, snapper, trout, tuna	Needed for energy metabolism
Potassium	Cod, halibut, perch, salmon, scallops, snapper, trout, tuna	Helps transmit nerve impulses, controls muscle contractions, and regulates water balance in tissue and cells
Magnesium	Mackerel, oysters, salmon, shrimp	Regulates heartbeat and promotes bone growth
Selenium	Cod, crab, lobster, oysters, scallops, shrimp	An important antioxidant that protects body cells from free-radical damage
Zinc	Crab, lobster, oysters, halibut	Aids in wound healing, growth, and sexual development

There are countless ways to enjoy fish and shellfish—especially when you follow the example of Mediterranean and Asian cultures that have spent thousands of years developing tasty recipes with fish and shellfish in the starring role. And because fish and shellfish cook very quickly, this also means you'll end up spending far less time in the kitchen than if you prepare a typical meat-based meal.

Following are some examples of different types of fish and shellfish and how you can easily incorporate them into your diet.

Anchovies. The salty flavor and oily texture of anchovies make them the classic complement for a wide variety of Mediterranean-style dishes. Sprinkle them over a pizza just before baking, add them to pasta sauces and risottos, and use them whole or finely chopped in Mediterranean-style salads. They also go wonderfully with a little chopped fresh basil as a topping for *bruschetta* (Italian garlic and olive oil toasts).

Clams. Clams add a delicious "taste of the sea" to pasta dishes, rice dishes, stews, and chowders. Canned clams can also be sprinkled on top of pizzas before baking.

Crab. Fresh crab is utterly delicious, but we regard it as "special occasion" food, because it's expensive and often hard to come by. More often than not we'll use surimi (imitation crab made from fish) instead. Whether you use real or imitation crab, either way you'll find plenty of uses for this versatile food. It can be added to stir-fries and noodle dishes; it tastes wonderful in risottos and pasta dishes, scattered in salads, or used as a filling in sushi, sandwiches, and rice-paper rolls.

Oysters and mussels. Smoked oysters and mussels can be used as a pizza topping or as part of an Italian *antipasto* platter. Fresh mussels in the shell are also as an important element in the classic Spanish seafood paella (a saffron-infused rice and vegetable dish studded with a variety of seafood). Fresh mussels also taste wonderful in pasta dishes and risottos. Oysters served raw in the shell with a little lemon juice make a delicious appetizer, but be sure that the oysters are really fresh and come from a reputable source.

Salmon. Salmon isn't only one of the richest sources of healthy omega-3s, it's also one of the most versatile varieties of fish:

Salmon steaks and salmon fillets: Salmon steaks are particularly good cooked over a hot grill and served with salad and crusty bread, but be careful not to overcook the delicate flesh or else it will dry out. Fresh salmon fillets can be grilled, steamed, poached with fresh herbs, marinated and baked, or cut into cubes and added to pasta dishes and stir-fries.

Smoked salmon: Thin slices of smoked salmon are delicious served with a bagel and a little cream cheese or avocado. Smoked salmon also makes a great pizza topping and sandwich or sushi filling, and it goes wonderfully with scrambled eggs.

Canned salmon: Canned salmon is ideal served cold with salad and bread or in a sandwich or sub. It also works equally well on pizzas and in pasta dishes, bakes, and risottos and can be used to make burger patties. Choose canned Alaskan red salmon, since this is the best quality.

Raw salmon: Very fresh raw salmon can be eaten Japanese-style, in sushi or thinly sliced and served as sashimi.

Sardines. Available fresh or canned. The canned variety can be mashed and used as a sandwich or toast spread, and the fresh variety goes well in pasta dishes or marinated and grilled.

Scallops. With their delicate milky flesh and clean flavor, scallops lend themselves to a wide variety of dishes including stir-fries, curries, pasta dishes, and bakes. Marinated and grilled scallops also make a delightful meal served with crusty bread and salad.

Shrimp. Shrimp happens to be one of our favorite foods. The possibilities with shrimp are virtually limitless: skewered with fresh vegetables, marinated, then cooked over a flaming grill; stir-fried with a colorful range of crunchy vegetables and served over rice or noodles; dotted throughout pasta dishes, risottos, pilafs, and paellas; as a filling for sandwiches and subs; or simply served as a classic shrimp cocktail with juicy tomatoes, crisp lettuce, tangy seafood sauce, and wedges of lemon. If you can't get your hands on fresh shrimp, frozen cooked shrimp is available in most supermarkets.

Squid.
Squid goes well in Mediterranean-style dishes like pasta, risotto, and pizza. It goes equally well with Asian-style dishes such as stir-fries, noodle dishes, and Asian braises.

Swordfish.
Swordfish is a delicious firm-fleshed fish with a mild flavor and a meaty texture. It's similar to fresh tuna and can be used in much the same way (see tuna below).

Tuna.
Like salmon, tuna is a good source of omega-3s and is incredibly versatile. And even if you're not a big fan of fish, you'll probably still enjoy tuna because its texture is more like chicken than fish.

Fresh tuna steaks are ideal grilled or panfried and served with salad and crusty bread. Fresh tuna can also be cut into cubes and added to pasta dishes, stews, curries, and stir-fries. Another way to enjoy fresh tuna is served raw in sushi and sashimi. Canned tuna is a staple food in our pantry and can be used in a myriad of wonderful dishes including pastas, pizzas, risottos, and bakes. Of course, canned tuna is also the ideal sandwich filing with fresh, crisp salad vegetables and a drizzle of mayo. We also use canned tuna to make our own "meaty" patties for burgers.

Whitefish.
Firm whitefish such as snapper, cod, and haddock can be cut into cubes and stir-fried, added to pasta dishes, or grilled or panfried whole with a little olive oil and served with freshly ground pepper and lemon juice. Whitefish of any kind also tastes wonderful marinated and baked or cooked in an Indian, Thai, or Malaysian curry until the flesh is soft and flaky.

Fish and shellfish are delicious, low in calories, easy to prepare, quick to cook, and incredibly versatile. And with all the wonderful health-giving benefits fish and other seafood have to offer, it's clear that including more in your diet (particularly in place of red meat) is a very sensible route to take. As Dr. Joyce A. Nettleton, a nutritionist and lecturer from Tufts University, Boston, puts it: "The benefits of including fish at least every week is no longer doubted . . . helping ourselves to fish is helping ourselves to health."

Plant Power

Plant-based foods form the backbone of traditional Mediterranean and Asian cuisine. One look at the Mediterranean and Asian Diet Pyramids (page 7) and this becomes very obvious. The typical Western way of eating, on the other hand, generally includes lots of meat and highly processed foods but usually very little fresh or minimally processed plant foods.

As more and more scientific studies point to the role that plant foods play in the promotion of health and the reduction of disease, this situation is slowly starting to change. But unfortunately most of us in the West still fall short in our consumption of plant foods.

Yet incorporating more plant foods into your diet is actually very easy to do. This chapter will show you how, by following the examples of Mediterranean and Asian cultures, eating more plant foods can actually be a highly pleasurable experience! This chapter will also identify the key reasons why you need to eat plant foods regularly if you want to give yourself the best chance of living a long and healthy life.

I've divided this chapter into four main sections. Each of these different types of plant foods has distinctive health-giving qualities, which I'll cover in detail.

Grain foods

Vegetables and fruits

Legumes

Nuts and seeds

COMMON TYPES OF GRAINS

- Wheat (used to make bread, pasta, noodles, couscous, and bulgur)

- Rice (comes in many different varieties and is eaten as a grain by itself or ground into rice flour to make various types of rice noodles)

- Oats

- Corn

- Rye

- Buckwheat (not botanically a grain but has a similar nutritional profile and is used in the same way)

- Barley

- Millet

GRAIN FOODS

For thousands of years, grain-based foods such as rice, bread, pasta, noodles, couscous, and bulgur have held a revered and sacred status throughout Asia and the Mediterranean. And it's not surprising that grains are so highly regarded by the peoples of these regions, because they really are an extraordinary food. They're inexpensive, filling, satisfying, and low in calories, and they can be used as a base for an almost endless variety of meals.

Grain foods are also highly nutritious. Wheat, for example, contains twenty-two different vitamins and minerals, including vitamin E and B1, niacin, folate, iron, zinc, selenium, potassium, and magnesium. Grain foods are also a good source of *antioxidants* and *phytochemicals*, which help promote good health and prevent disease. (I'll talk more about these incredible substances later in this chapter.) And like all plant foods, grains—particularly whole grains—are a good source of health-promoting *dietary fiber* (see "Dietary Fiber and Its Benefits," page 38).

Studies have even found that whole grains can protect against heart disease and cancer. In one study, researchers from the University of Minnesota studied nearly 34,000 people and found that those who ate the highest amount of whole grains had a 23 percent reduced risk of death from heart disease and a 21 percent reduced risk of death from cancer when compared with people who ate little or no whole grains.

DIETARY FIBER AND ITS BENEFITS

Dietary fiber is a type of carbohydrate found only in plant foods. It's basically derived from the material that helps give plants their shape and structure. Fiber falls into two distinct categories: insoluble fiber and soluble fiber. Most plant foods contain a combination of both soluble and insoluble fiber in varying amounts.

Insoluble fiber, which is found in high amounts in whole grains as well as beans, fruits, and vegetables, is coarse in texture. Soluble fiber, on the other hand, has a soft and gummy texture and is found in high amounts in legumes (beans, peas, and lentils), fruits, vegetables, oats, and barley. Soluble and insoluble fiber work in different ways to promote health.

Insoluble Fiber

Insoluble fiber acts like a sponge and absorbs water as it's digested, so it adds bulk and softness to bowel movements. This not only prevents constipation, but also speeds the rate at which food passes through your system, leaving less time for certain foods to deposit impurities and cancer-promoting compounds on the intestinal wall. This may be one reason why diets high in fiber are associated with low rates of bowel and colon cancer. Recent results from one of the largest studies ever conducted into the link between diet and cancer—the EPIC (European Prospective Investigation of Cancer and Nutrition) Study—involving more than 500,000 people from ten countries for nearly five years, found that the people eating the most fiber had a 40 percent lower risk of colon cancer than those people eating the least.

Soluble Fiber

Soluble fiber works differently from insoluble fiber because it's broken down by the action of bacteria in the digestive tract and some of the healthy by-products of this process are absorbed into the bloodstream. Once in the bloodstream, these healthy by-products have been found to bind with bile acids (compounds originally derived from cholesterol stores in the liver) and escort them out of the body. This draws cholesterol from the blood and in turn lowers cholesterol levels. In one study of men with high cholesterol levels, adding half a cup of cooked dried beans (rich in soluble fiber) to their normal diet reduced their blood cholesterol levels by 13 percent in twenty-one days. Soluble fiber also slows the release of glucose into the bloodstream, which helps regulate blood sugar levels.

Both soluble and insoluble fibers have also been shown to protect against heart disease and breast cancer. A study of more than 43,000 U.S. male health professionals, conducted by Harvard University, found that over a six-year period those who ate the most fiber had a 55 percent lower chance of coronary death than those who ate the least. And a recent study of more than 1,000 Australian women (half had been diagnosed with breast cancer, half were free of the disease) found that those who ate more than 28 grams of fiber per day had the lowest risk of the disease, while those who ate less than 14 grams per day faced the highest risk.

The Weight-Loss Bonus

Fiber not only promotes good health and keeps you regular, but it can also help control your weight. Here's why. First, fiber is nature's best appetite suppressant, because it fills the stomach and satisfies your appetite much earlier than fiber-depleted foods. And fiber isn't only bulky and filling; it also can't be digested like normal foods (it basically passes right through you), so it adds virtually no calories to your diet.

The chewiness of high-fiber foods also prolongs eating time, which, in turn, gives your body time to tell your brain that your stomach is full.

And a high-fiber diet may actually cut the number of calories you ingest by blocking your body's ability to digest the fat and protein consumed along with it. In a recent study by the U.S. Department of Agriculture, researchers set a certain number of calories for subject groups and altered the fiber content. Results demonstrated that fewer calories were absorbed with increased fiber intake. It was found that people who consumed up to 36 grams of fiber a day absorbed 130 fewer daily calories. Over a year that adds up to more than 47,000 calories!

Are You Getting Enough?

The importance of fiber as part of a healthy diet is beyond question. Unfortunately, most people in Western countries, like the United States, the United Kingdom, and Australia, consume very little dietary fiber—only around 10 to 15 grams a day. While this is better than none, it's too little for any appreciable benefit. Throughout the Mediterranean and Asia, fiber intake is traditionally between 30 and 40 grams a day. This is the level to strive for. Luckily, by following a MediterrAsian style of eating—which includes lots of fiber-rich whole grains, fruits, vegetables, nuts, and legumes—you'll naturally be eating this level of fiber without having to think about it.

To many people's surprise, grains are also a good source of protein. Most varieties of grain contain 10 to 15 percent protein. However, unlike fish, soybeans, and meat, this protein isn't "complete" because it's low in *lysine* (one of the amino acids, or building blocks, of protein). But this problem is easily overcome by mixing a grain food with a complementary protein that contains *lysine*, such as legumes (beans, peas, and lentils), nuts, or fish. Indeed, this is what Mediterraneans and Asians have instinctively been doing for centuries.

Grains and Carbohydrates

Ever wondered how Chinese peasants or Greek farmers can toil away in the fields for long hours every day, even well into old age? Part of the answer could lie in the energy-giving foods these people eat every day.

Traditional Mediterranean and Asian diets are based on a foundation of grain foods like rice, bread, pasta, and noodles. These foods also happen to contain plenty of energy-giving carbohydrates. All plant foods, including beans, vegetables, and fruits, contain carbohydrates; however, grain foods are one of the richest sources.

The reason why carbohydrates are so good at boosting energy levels is simple: when they're digested, they're broken down in your body and converted into glucose, or what is commonly known as blood sugar. This glucose is then released into your bloodstream, and it supplies your muscles with their favorite source of fuel. So, by regularly eating carbohydrate-rich grain foods, you'll always ensure your energy levels stay high.

Just think, the grain-rich diets of the Mediterranean region and Asia are what helped fuel the conquering Roman legions, sustained the laborers as they built the Great Pyramids, and provided the energy for the workers to build the Great Wall of China. Imagine how this same type of diet can help power you through your day!

Brain Fuel

The glucose supplied by carbohydrates isn't the favorite source of fuel for only your muscles: Your brain runs almost exclusively on glucose. That's why, if your blood sugar levels get low, you feel not only low in energy but often moody and fuzzy-headed, and it becomes difficult to concentrate. And carbohydrates have another important effect on the brain—they naturally increase the production of *serotonin*, a special chemical in the brain that has a calming effect.

So, by eating plenty of carbohydrates, you'll be more mentally alert and focused throughout the day, and at the same time you should also feel calmer and less moody.

Regulating Blood Sugars

Carbohydrate-rich grain foods are great for supplying your muscles and brain with glucose. However, to ensure this glucose is delivered most effectively, it makes sense to mix grain foods with foods that contain fat and protein. This is because fat and protein help to slow down the release of glucose into your bloodstream, which in turn helps regulate your blood sugars. (Soluble fiber, found in high amounts in legumes, vegetables, and fruits, also slows down the release of glucose into the bloodstream.)

This slow and steady release of glucose ensures you'll have a constant supply of fuel for your muscles and brain, which ultimately means more energy for longer periods of time, better concentration, and fewer mood swings.

The great thing is that grain-based foods like pasta and rice taste much better with the addition of protein and fat anyway. In fact, Mediterranean and Asian peoples have traditionally been mixing grain foods with protein sources (such as fish, beans, and poultry) and fat (such as olive oil and peanut oil) for thousands of years. Later in the book we'll show you just how easy it is to mix your meals in the same way (see page 94).

White or Whole Grain?

When it comes to buying grain-based foods, you'll find there are two distinct categories: white and whole grain (also known as whole wheat or wholemeal). White or whole-grain pasta, white or brown (whole-grain) rice, and white or whole-grain bread are some examples.

What's the difference between the white and whole-grain varieties? Well, whole grains are just that—the whole grain. An unrefined kernel of grain is actually made up of three layers: the germ (innermost layer), the endosperm (central core), and the bran (protective outer layer). Refined (white) grains, on the other hand, have had their bran and germ removed in the refining process. Although the germ and bran layers make up less than 20 percent of the actual volume of a kernel of grain, two-thirds of the fiber and many of the vitamins and minerals are located in these layers.

So, nutritionally speaking, white grain products are inferior to whole-grain products. But does this make white grain products unhealthy? Well, think about it this way. If you took an apple and peeled it, would the apple suddenly become unhealthy? Sure, a peeled apple won't be as good for you as an unpeeled apple, because lots of fiber, vitamins, and minerals are stored in the skin of the apple; but this doesn't make what's left unhealthy.

The same is true with grains. White grain foods may not be as healthy for you as whole-grain foods, but they're certainly not an unhealthy food. What is left when the germ and bran has been removed is the endosperm, or central core of the grain, which contains energy-giving carbohydrates as well as protein and B vitamins. And the endosperm still contains a third of the health-promoting fiber found in a grain's kernel.

So, white grain products aren't bad for you at all (unless they're combined with sugar or bad fats or cooked with unhealthy ingredients) and should definitely have a place in your diet. In fact, in most parts of Asia and the Mediterranean region, white rice and pasta have been more popular than whole-grain varieties for many generations.

At the same time, it's clear that whole grains are very important because of the valuable nutrients they provide. The solution? Eat regular pasta and rice, and when it comes to breads and breakfast cereals, opt mostly for whole-grain varieties. This way you'll ensure you get a rich mix of nutrients.

Fitting Grain Foods into Your Life

With all the benefits that grain foods have to offer, it's now a matter of incorporating more of them into your life so you can reap the rewards. Luckily this is easily accomplished because a MediterrAsian style of eating features grain foods in a prominent role (as you'll discover when you try the delicious recipes in this book). Here's a rundown of the most common types of grain foods you'll be eating as part of a MediterrAsian way of eating.

Rice. The Chinese eat the most rice in the world, at over four pounds (uncooked weight) per person each week. With this in mind, it's probably not surprising that the Chinese word for rice, *fan*, means "food." Rice is also a staple food in most other Asian countries, including Japan, Thailand, Indonesia, Vietnam, and India.

But rice isn't popular only in Asia—for centuries it has also been widely enjoyed throughout the Mediterranean. The peoples of the Mediterranean have put their own flare into this versatile food and some of the delicious rice dishes popular in these regions include *risotto* from Italy, *paella* from Spain, and *pilaf* from Greece and the Middle East.

In recent years Western consumers have started to realize the benefits of this inexpensive and healthy grain. These days there are many varieties of rice available at your local supermarket. Some examples include fragrant Thai *jasmine*, Indian *basmati*, Spanish *valencia*, Japanese *koshihikari* (ideal for sushi), and Italian *arborio* (perfect for risottos).

Pasta. Pasta has been a staple food in the Italian diet for centuries. As far back as 1300 the ships of Genoa had a "master of lasagna" on board to cook for the sailors.

And there are so many reasons to love pasta: It's quick and easy to prepare, inexpensive, incredibly versatile, moderate in calories (a one-cup serving of cooked pasta contains only around 190 calories), and above all else it tastes delicious!

Pasta can be made from rice, corn, buckwheat, and other grains, but typically it's made from wheat, preferably durum wheat (a special hard type of wheat that's ideal for pasta making). You can buy pasta fresh, dried, and in high-fiber whole-grain varieties.

Much of the appeal of pasta lies in its sheer versatility. Not only are the topping ideas limited only by your imagination, but the range of pasta shapes and sizes is enormous, with more than four hundred different varieties. Some of our favorites include spaghetti, lasagna, fusilli (corkscrew shape), fettuccine (flat, rib-bonlike), penne (tubular with ends cut on diagonal), farfalle (bow-tie shaped), cappellini (angel hair), and conchiglie (shells). One of the delights of eating a pasta dish is determining by experiment which kind of pasta best matches your favorite sauces.

Noodles.

Born in China around four thousand years ago, noodles are to Asians what pasta is to Italians. This endlessly versatile food can be boiled and served with sauces and toppings, simmered in soups and braises, or stir-fried with thinly sliced vegetables, seafood, and meats.

Noodles are commonly made from wheat or rice flour, but other varieties are available made from buckwheat or bean starch. Depending on their shape and size, most noodles take only 5 to 10 minutes to cook.

Although noodles are generally low in calories, some varieties (like instant ramen noodles) contain a fairly large amount of fat in the form of palm oil. Unfortunately, palm oil is as highly saturated as animal fat, and so its use should be limited. Instead, look for noodles that contain just flour and water, since these are the healthiest option.

Bread.

Bread, which has often been referred to as "the staff of life," is one of the most widely consumed foods in the world. In the Mediterranean region, where bread originated more than four thousand years ago, it's a staple food that's eaten at most meals.

Bread is also a popular food in the West, but many of us tend to limit our choice of bread to sliced white. This is unfortunate, because there is such a vast range of alternative breads available, offering a world of tastes and textures. Some examples include Italian ciabatta and focaccia bread, baguettes, pita bread, whole-grain peasant bread, Turkish *pide* bread, Middle Eastern lavash bread, Indian naan bread, as well as a large range of specialty loaves and rolls. Experiment with different breads to find your favorites.

Couscous and bulgur.

Both of these grain foods are actually made from wheat. Couscous is made from durum wheat (the same type of wheat used to make pasta), which is moistened with water, then rolled in small balls and steamed. It's a staple food in the north African countries that border the Mediterranean Sea, including Morocco and Tunisia, and it is traditionally served topped with various kinds of vegetable, fish, poultry, and bean stews. Couscous can also be added to salads, used to thicken soups, or mixed with fruit and other ingredients to make wonderful sweet desserts.

Bulgur is made from whole wheat that has been parboiled, dried, then sifted into particles. Bulgur is a common food in Greece and the countries of the Middle East, and like couscous it can be topped with various kinds of stews and sauces or used to thicken soups. It's also delicious used in pilafs and is an important ingredient in tabbouleh salad.

Breakfast cereals.

Breakfast cereals fit in perfectly with a Mediterr-Asian way of eating because they're made from grains such as wheat, oats, and rice. With a little milk and topped with some fruit, breakfast cereals make an ideal high-energy start to the day.

Of course, all breakfast cereals aren't created equal, and many have a lot of added sugar, salt, and hydrogenated fats. The cereals to look out for are the whole-grain varieties because these not only have more fiber but often contain little or no added nasties (oatmeal and untoasted muesli are ideal).

And don't think of breakfast cereals as something to have just at breakfast. They also make a great anytime snack and are a particularly good substitute for less nutritious snacks like chips and candy.

VEGETABLES AND FRUITS

More than two thousand years ago, the Greek physician Hippocrates proclaimed: "Let food be your medicine, and medicine be your food." Over the last few decades scientific research has proven just how true are Hippocrates' words of wisdom. Many types of foods are now known to contain nutrients that act like medicine and improve health and that also reduce the risk of becoming ill in the first place. Vegetables and fruits, more than any other types of food, contain the widest range of health-promoting compounds, including antioxidants, phytochemicals, soluble and insoluble fibers, and a host of essential vitamins and minerals.

A large body of research in recent years has shown that these compounds can help your body resist cancer, heart disease, and other chronic health conditions. Vegetables and fruits are also generally very low in saturated fat and calories, incredibly versatile, and when prepared correctly taste great.

Notice how I say *when prepared correctly* they taste great. Because when vegetables and fruits—particularly vegetables—aren't prepared properly they can taste very unappetizing, to say the least. And that's probably one of the main reasons why vegetables aren't particularly popular in Western society—we really don't know how to prepare them properly.

Enjoying Vegetables

Remember the "eat your vegetables" routine at the dinner table? I certainly do; often followed by the threat that if I didn't my dessert would instead be given to my older sister. And it's through similar threats and bribes that many of us were forced to eat vegetables as kids, and unfortunately a lot of us have grown up to hate vegetables as adults.

But compare this to people living in Mediterranean and Asian countries like Italy, Japan, Greece, or China; for thousands of years they've never had a problem eating and enjoying their vegetables. Why? Because the traditional way Mediterranean and Asian peoples prepare and serve vegetables is very different from how we do it in the West and vastly more appetizing.

In the West we often treat vegetables like a separate part of the meal and have them unflavored and pushed off into the corner of our plate. Throughout the Mediterranean region and Asia, on the other hand, vegetables are rarely served in a pile by themselves. Vegetables are an integral part of the taste, texture, and color of most traditional Mediterranean and Asian dishes, and they're typically cut up and mixed in and cooked with the rest of the meal. And it's by combining vegetables with grain foods and protein-rich foods (like fish, shellfish, beans, and chicken), as well as sauces and flavorings, that vegetables taste their best.

Actually, we really already know this in the West, because a well-made sandwich is based on the same principle. If you munched away on plain lettuce or tomato you'd soon get bored; but when tomatoes and lettuce are combined with bread (grain food) and some tuna or chicken (protein-rich food) and some mustard or mayo (flavoring), you suddenly have a tasty sandwich. Indeed, the sandwich wouldn't taste as good without the crunchy lettuce and juicy tomatoes.

And that's the secret to enjoying vegetables: not having them plain and unflavored on the side of your plate but using them as an integral part of your meal. Thankfully this is easy to do because generations of home cooks from the Mediterranean region and Asia have developed countless mouthwatering dishes that use vegetables as a major component. Some good examples include stir-fries, curries, pizzas, pasta dishes, risottos, pilafs, and paellas.

Enjoying Fruit

Fruit also plays a very important role in traditional Mediterranean and Asian diets, and it is typically eaten daily as a snack and dessert.

In Western society, although fruit is generally thought of in a more kindly way than are vegetables, again we don't eat nearly as much as we should. A recent study in the United States found that nearly half of all Americans eat no fruit on a given day, and there have been similar findings in the United Kingdom, Australia, New Zealand, and Canada.

There seem to be two major reasons why we don't eat very much fresh fruit in modern Western society. For a start, when was the last time you saw an advertisement for fresh fruit? Yet when was the last time you saw an advertisement for fruit's biggest rival, candy and processed desserts?

Not helping the situation is the fact that the Western way with fruits also tends to be rather unimaginative. For example, many of us limit our choice of fruit to apples, oranges, and a small handful of other fruits. But even though apples and oranges taste delicious, there are dozens of other equally delicious fruits to choose from. Let your imagination run wild when it comes to choosing fruit—mangoes, pineapple, kiwi fruit, berries (strawberries, raspberries, and so on), grapes, lychees, passion fruit, melons (watermelon, cantaloupe, and the like), papaya, persimmons, plums, figs, apricots, and cherries are just some delicious examples. And be adventurous with the way you eat fruits. As well as eating them by themselves, cut them up and mix different fruits together to create a varied range of fruit salads and fruit platters.

Fruit also makes a great base for lots of wonderful, healthy desserts and smoothies. Fresh or dried fruit can also add a sweet accent to savory salads, and it makes a particularly good breakfast-cereal topper.

Another way you can enjoy fruit is to lighten up a rich dessert. Instead of having a whole serving of rich dessert, have half a serving and mix it with pieces of fresh fruit of your choice. This will add wonderful color, texture, and taste to the dessert, as well as lower the overall calories. We enjoy putting this principle into practice regularly by having fresh fruit salad with a scoop of our favorite ice cream.

The Health-Giving Powers of Vegetables and Fruits

The examples above give you some good ideas of how to include more vegetables and fruits in your diet. And it's certainly not just your taste buds that will benefit. As I mentioned earlier, vegetables and fruits have extraordinary disease-fighting powers. An increasing body of scientific evidence dramatically highlights this protective effect.

The *Journal of the American Medical Association*, for example, recently reported on findings from a long-term study of more than eight hundred middle-aged men from Framingham, Massachusetts. The study found that the men who ate the most vegetables and fruits were the least likely to have had a stroke. For every three servings eaten a day, researchers found the risk of stroke dropped 22 percent. Two large-scale studies by researchers at Harvard School of Public Health and Brigham and Women's Hospital in Boston also found that eating plenty of vegetables and fruits offers protection against stroke. Both studies found that eating five servings of vegetables and fruits a day was associated with a 30-percent lower risk of stroke for men and women.

To date more than three hundred studies have also found that vegetables and fruits protect against different types of cancer. These include most of the cancers common in Western society, such as breast, prostate, colon, and lung cancer.

In a major study published in the *Journal of the American Dietetic Association,* researchers from the United States and Germany reviewed more than two hundred of these studies. They found consistent evidence that people who ate plenty of vegetables and fruits (five or more servings a day) had about half the risk of developing a broad range of cancers compared with people who ate few vegetables and fruits.

More than twenty studies have also shown that vegetables and fruits protect against heart disease. One study in Finland that tracked more than 5,000 Finnish men and women for fourteen years found that the one-third of study participants who ate the most vegetables and fruit had a 34 percent reduction in the risk of a fatal heart attack when compared with the one-third eating the least vegetables and fruit.

Vegetables and fruits have even been found to offer protection against the bone-thinning disease osteoporosis. A study by researchers at Tufts University in Boston found that a high intake of vegetables and fruits helped determine the strength and density of bones in old age.

The lead investigator of the study, Katherine L. Tucker, PhD, associate professor of nutrition at Tufts University, reported: "This suggests that a good quality diet in adulthood is important to bone health beyond the better known contributions of calcium and vitamin D, and provides yet another reason to emphasize the intake of fruits and vegetables."

When you combine this sort of evidence with the fact that the vegetable- and fruit-loving peoples of the Mediterranean region and Asia also have low rates of these same diseases, it becomes pretty clear that an apple a day really does keep the doctor away.

Nutrient Rich, Calorie Poor

Vegetables and fruits may be nutrient rich, but they're also calorie poor. In other words, vegetables and fruits give you the biggest bang for the buck—lots of nutrients for the lowest amount of calories.

Did you know, for example, that two quarter-pound cheeseburgers contain the same number of calories as fifty carrots or seventy tomatoes?

Of course, I don't expect you to sit down to a plate of seventy tomatoes for lunch tomorrow, but this comparison gives you a good idea that when you add lots of different vegetables and fruits to your diet, you'll be adding lots of taste, texture, flavor, color, and nutrients but very few calories.

And the reason is quite simple: Vegetables and fruits generally have a very high water content. Because water contains no calories, vegetables and fruits, in turn, contain very few calories.

As an added bonus, the calories in vegetables and fruits generally come from carbohydrates, which are broken down into glucose in your body. Because glucose provides fuel for your muscles to work, it makes it much easier to incorporate more activity into your life, which in itself burns calories.

Vegetables and fruits are also a good source of dietary fiber. Fiber fills you up without filling you out, and because it can't be digested it adds virtually no calories to your diet.

However, not all vegetables and fruits are the same. When fresh vegetables or fruits are dried or turned into juice, the process changes their concentration of calories. In the case of fruit and vegetable juice, the calories become more concentrated because most of the fiber and bulk have been removed. Dried fruit, on the other hand, contains a much higher concentration of calories than fresh fruit because most of the water has been removed.

Removing the fiber or water from fruits and vegetables not only concentrates calories but also makes them less bulky and not as filling and satisfying. This was clearly demonstrated in a study by Dr. Kenneth Heaton and colleagues at Bristol University, England. They gave ten volunteers either a whole apple or the same amount of apple made into puree or into juice. The volunteers took, on average, seventeen minutes to eat the apple, six minutes to eat the puree, and only one and a half minutes to drink the juice. Predictably, the volunteers said that the whole apples were more satisfying and kept them fuller for much longer.

Of course, juiced or dried vegetables and fruits are fine in moderation, but the most satisfying and certainly the healthiest way to eat vegetables and fruits is in their natural, "whole" state.

All vegetables and fruits contain health-giving powers to a certain extent, but researchers have identified a number of vegetables and fruits that are particularly beneficial. Not surprisingly, all of these vegetables and fruits happen to be eaten extensively throughout Asia and the Mediterranean region.

Garlic

A classic ingredient in traditional Mediterranean and Asian cooking, garlic has long been regarded as one of nature's most effective cure-alls. As long ago as 3000 BC, Egyptians were worshipping garlic and using it as a medicine (clay models of garlic were found inside Tutankhamen's tomb). Traditional Chinese medicine used garlic for the treatment of coughs, colds, bronchitis, tuberculosis, diarrhea, and many other infectious diseases. The ancient Greek physician Hippocrates used garlic to treat certain cancers. And it has been used throughout history to treat a host of other ailments including the plague in Europe and typhus and dysentery during World War I.

Since the 1950s, dozens of scientific studies have evaluated the health and healing powers of garlic, and a number of other benefits have been discovered. Donald D. Hensrud, MD, a nutrition specialist at the Mayo Clinic in Minnesota notes: "Research is concentrating on several areas where garlic may have positive effects: cardiovascular health, immune function, antimicrobial action and anticancer activity."

In a recent study of 42,000 women in Iowa, for example, those who ate garlic more than once a week were half as likely to develop colon cancer as those who did not eat garlic. Garlic has also been shown to lower LDL (bad) cholesterol and boost HDL (good) cholesterol, which can decrease the incidence of heart attack and stroke.

So what makes garlic such a powerful superfood? Researchers have found that garlic is full of health-giving compounds, including vitamin C, potassium, phosphorus, selenium, and a number of amino acids. But one of the most important health-giving compounds found in garlic is allicin, a phytochemical compound formed when garlic is cut or crushed (it's allicin that gives garlic its characteristic flavor and pungent aroma).

Garlic is enjoyed daily throughout the Mediterranean region, and it is used as a flavor enhancer in pasta dishes, paellas, risottos, pilafs, pizzas, stews, soups, salad dressings, and sauces. Garlic is an equally essential ingredient in Asian cooking. "The pungent flavor of garlic is part of the fabric of Chinese cuisine," points out renowned Chinese American cook and author Ken Hom. "It would be inconceivable to cook without its distinctive, highly aromatic smell and unique taste."

continues on next page

Tomatoes

Tomatoes are a staple ingredient in Mediterranean cooking (they were brought back from the New World by Spanish explorers around five hundred years ago), and they are also popular in Indian and Southeast Asian cooking.

The unique flavor and texture of tomatoes complement a multitude of dishes, including hearty stews, robust pasta dishes, spicy curries, and mouthwatering soups (such as Italian minestrone and Spanish gazpacho). Many types of salad also rely on the juiciness, flavor, and color of tomatoes, including Greek salad, and Salade Niçoise. And, of course, pizza wouldn't be quite the same without a layer of luscious tomato sauce.

But tomatoes aren't renowned only for their taste and versatility; research in recent years has found that tomatoes also act as a potent medicine. And the characteristic deep red color of tomatoes is one of the reasons they're so healthy. It turns out that the pigment that gives tomatoes their color—called lycopene—has powerful antioxidant properties and also protects against cancer. Research has shown that lycopene is particularly effective at reducing the risk of prostate cancer. In a large-scale study by Harvard researchers involving more than 48,000 men, it was found that those who ate ten or more servings of lycopene-rich tomato products a week had one-third the risk of developing prostate cancer than those eating two servings or fewer a week. A review of more than seventy studies published in the *Journal of the National Cancer Institute* also found strong evidence that lycopene protects against prostate cancer, as well as lung and stomach cancers.

And lycopene doesn't offer protection against only cancer. A study involving 1,300 European men found that those consuming the most lycopene from foods had about half the risk of heart attack as men who consumed the least.

Along with lycopene, tomatoes are also rich in vitamin C and beta-carotene (both powerful antioxidants), and they are a good source of health-promoting dietary fiber and potassium. To top it off, tomatoes are also very low in calories.

Berries

Berries are sweet and satisfying superfoods. Strawberries, cranberries, raspberries, and blackberries are all packed with powerful antioxidants and phytochemicals that ward off disease and premature aging. Berries also supply your body with a host of other essential nutrients, including potassium, vitamin C, iron, B vitamins such as niacin (which releases energy from food and protects against heart disease), and folate.

Raspberries and strawberries are two of the richest food sources of a phytochemical compound called *ellagic acid*, which studies have shown to be a powerful cancer blocker. Cranberries and blueberries contain antibiotic-like compounds that help prevent bladder and urinary tract infection. And all berries contain high amounts of pectin, a soluble fiber that has been shown to be effective at lowering blood-cholesterol levels by binding with cholesterol and eliminating it from the body.

There are plenty of ways to enjoy berries: sprinkled over cereals, added to fruit salads, whipped up in a smoothie, served with a scoop of your favorite ice cream, or simply eaten by themselves as a sweet and juicy snack.

Avocados

Avocados are one of the few fruits that are high in fat. But unlike saturated fat, which can raise potentially harmful LDL-cholesterol levels in your body, the fat in avocados is mostly made up of heart-healthy monounsaturated fat. Avocados also contain high amounts of special phytochemical compounds called *phytosterols*. Studies have shown that phytosterols can inhibit cholesterol absorption from the intestine, which results in lower levels of LDL cholesterol in the blood. In animal studies, phytosterols have also been shown to inhibit the growth of cancerous tumors.

In addition, avocados are a rich source of vitamin E, a powerful antioxidant that protects your cells from free-radical damage. They also contain high amounts of folate, which has been shown to protect against heart disease as well as to prevent birth defects. And avocados are also one of the richest sources of the mineral potassium, which helps to maintain the stability of heart cells and the central nervous system.

But, although avocados are very healthy, it's important to remember that they're also very high in calories (one medium-size avocado contains around 500 calories), so it makes sense not to go overboard when you eat them. Luckily, because they're so rich and creamy, a little avocado goes a long way. Use them diced into salads and sandwiches, blend them up with some lemon juice and salt for an instant guacamole dip, or try them Japanese style in sushi rolls with smoked salmon or shrimp. A particularly good way to enjoy avocados is as a healthy alternative to butter. Simply mash some avocado in a cup or bowl, and smear it onto your sandwich before you add the fillings.

Cruciferous Vegetables

I was put off the cruciferous family very early in life when my mother introduced me to brussels sprouts. They were usually served overcooked and soggy and were always the last thing on my plate to get eaten. Thankfully I'm now on good terms with the cruciferous family, because I've discovered that when they're cooked the right way (the MediterrAsian way, of course), they can taste absolutely delicious! Here are some choices from this varied vegetable group:

continues on next page

Bok choy	Choy sum
Broccoli	Gai lan
Brussels sprouts	Mustard greens
Cabbage	Rutabaga
Cauliflower	Swiss chard
Chinese cabbage	

Yet again the home cooks of the Mediterranean region and Asia have come up with a delightful array of ways to use these vegetables to add flavor, depth, and texture to a wide range of wonderful dishes from soups, salads, and stir-fries to curries, stews, and pasta dishes.

And the cruciferous family isn't only a tasty addition to a myriad of dishes. These vegetables also happen to be one of the most powerful disease-fighting plant foods known to science.

About twenty years ago studies first indicated that a high consumption of cruciferous vegetables equaled a reduced risk of certain cancers. Then in the early 1990s a phytochemical called *sulforaphane* was identified in cruciferous vegetables that was found to guard against cancer by stimulating the production of protective enzymes that detoxify carcinogens (cancer-causing compounds). In addition, another compound was discovered called *indol-3-carbinol*, which was found to reduce breast cancer risk by preventing estrogen overproduction. A Harvard study even found that a high intake of cruciferous vegetables, such as broccoli and cabbage, could reduce bladder cancer risk in men.

Cruciferous vegetables are also a rich source of many other potent disease-fighting substances, including potassium, calcium, and dietary fiber. And broccoli and cabbage are a good source of immune-system-boosting, antioxidant-rich vitamin C. For example, one medium stalk of broccoli provides 200 percent of the daily recommended intake of vitamin C.

Carrots

Remember being told that carrots helped you see better in the dark? Well, they do. Carrots are rich in *beta-carotene*, which is converted by the body into vitamin A, a nutrient essential for the functioning of your eyes' retinas.

Beta-carotene, which is a powerful antioxidant, has also been shown to improve immune function, inhibit the early stages of tumor development, and lower cholesterol levels. In one study, participants who ate seven carrots a day for three weeks dropped their cholesterol levels by 11 percent.

Carrots are also one of the best vegetable sources of health-giving dietary fiber, containing high amounts of both soluble and insoluble fiber.

Carrots make a colorful and crunchy addition to stir-fries and stews, and they taste wonderful finely chopped in pasta dishes, shredded on sandwiches, added to salads, or simply eaten raw as a snack.

Citrus Fruits

The citrus family includes oranges and lemons, which have been widely cultivated in the Mediterranean region since ancient Roman times; limes, which are native to India; and mandarins, which have been grown in China and Japan for thousands of years. Other citrus fruit include grapefruit, tangerines, and tangelos.

All citrus fruits are a good source of *flavonoids*—a special group of phytochemicals, which have been found to inhibit the growth of breast, prostate, and skin cancer cells. In addition, oranges and tangelos are rich sources of a phytochemical called *5-desmethyl sinensetin*, which has been shown to effectively inhibit human lung-cancer cells.

Citrus fruits, as we've always been told, are also a good source of vitamin C (one orange, for example, contains two times your daily requirement of vitamin C). Vitamin C not only works as a powerful free-radical-destroying antioxidant but also makes blood less likely to clot, which reduces the risk of heart attack and stroke. Citrus fruits also contain high amounts of a soluble fiber called *pectin*, which helps lower potentially harmful LDL blood-cholesterol levels.

Citrus fruits can be enjoyed in dozens of different ways. Oranges, tangelos, and tangerines can be eaten by themselves, juiced, or chopped and mixed in with other fruits to make a variety of fruit salads. Citrus fruits also go well as a sweet addition to savory salads. Lemon or lime juice and zest can be used as a flavor enhancer in a myriad of dishes such as curries, pasta dishes, and soups, and lemon juice or lime juice adds a delightful tang to salad dressings. Fresh lemon juice squeezed over fish and shellfish is also the perfect accompaniment.

Onions

Onions are related to garlic, and like garlic, onions are a staple in traditional Mediterranean and Asian cooking. Onions also share many of garlic's health-giving properties. They have been shown to boost good HDL-cholesterol levels while lowering potentially harmful LDL cholesterol. They increase blood-clot-dissolving activity in the blood, which reduces the risk of heart attack and stroke. And studies have identified a phytochemical in onions called *quercetin*, which is a powerful antioxidant and cancer-attacking agent.

Sautéed, chopped onions are used as the base for a wide variety of Mediterranean and Asian meals including risottos, curries, pasta dishes, pilafs, and paellas. Thinly sliced raw onion also adds a wonderful boost to salads, sandwiches, and burgers (red onions are particularly

continues on next page

good because they're milder, sweeter, and more colorful than regular onions). And when whole onions are roasted, they lose their potency and become sweet, delicate vegetables.

Bell Peppers

Bell peppers come in many colors—green, red, yellow, and even orange. Their color depends on the variety and their stage of ripeness.

Red peppers are particularly healthy because they are a rich source of the powerful antioxidants vitamin C and beta-carotene (red peppers contain around ten times more beta-carotene than green peppers). One 3½-ounce red pepper contains the recommended daily allowance of beta-carotene and more than 300 percent of the recommended daily allowance for vitamin C. And red peppers, like tomatoes, contain cancer-fighting lycopene.

Bell peppers can be enjoyed in many different ways, such as cut into thin strips and lightly cooked in stir-fries or cooked until melt-in-the-mouth tender in stews and pasta sauces. Roasted and marinated peppers also go wonderfully in an Italian antipasto platter or a Middle Eastern meze platter. And thinly sliced raw peppers make a crunchy and colorful addition to salads and sandwiches.

How to Easily Consume These Superfoods Regularly

When you eat the MediterrAsian way you'll find that most of your meals will contain at least one of the nine vegetables or fruits listed above, and often more. A stir-fry or pasta dish, for example, could easily contain garlic, onion, bell pepper, broccoli, and carrots. If you finish with a fresh fruit salad that includes berries and oranges, you've eaten seven different types in one sitting!

LEGUMES

For centuries legumes have played a major role in the traditional diets enjoyed by Mediterranean and Asian peoples. In the Tuscany region of Italy, for example, there is such a wide variety of bean dishes that Tuscans are fondly known as the "bean eaters." Throughout India, legumes such as chickpeas, lentils, and green peas form a cornerstone of many Indian curries, such as dahl (lentil curry). In Greece and the countries of the Middle East, beans and lentils are traditionally eaten daily in soups and stews or turned into sauces and pastes such as hummus. And in Asian countries, such as Japan and China, the soybean in its many forms—such as tofu and soy sauce—is an essential ingredient in traditional cooking.

But legumes aren't only a delicious base for countless tasty meals. In recent years scientists have discovered that legumes are also nutritional powerhouses containing many essential nutrients we need for good health from the cradle to the grave. In addition to being a nutritious food source, studies have shown that legumes can also help lower LDL-cholesterol levels, decrease the risk of certain cancers, help control diabetes, relieve symptoms of menopause (such as hot flashes and night sweats), and assist in weight maintenance.

A Health Jackpot

There are so many reasons why legumes are such a health-giving food. First, they are a valuable source of both carbohydrates and protein. Carbohydrates are your muscles' and brain's favorite fuel source, and protein is used by your body for growth and repair, so both of these nutrients are vital for good health. Legumes also contain high amounts of soluble fiber, which helps slow the rate at which glucose (blood sugar) enters your bloodstream—so you'll have more energy and better concentration for longer periods of time. The soluble fiber in legumes has also been shown to help lower blood-cholesterol levels.

In addition to carbohydrates, protein, and fiber, beans and other legumes are also a good source of zinc, phosphorus, magnesium, and potassium. These minerals are important for maintaining healthy muscle tone, combating fatigue, and promoting energy and endurance. Legumes are also a good source of iron (which helps deliver oxygen to all your cells) and B vitamins (which are important for a number of bodily functions, including maintaining healthy nerve cells and strengthening your immune system).

Meat for Vegetarians

Legumes have often been called "meat for vegetarians" and for a very good reason. Beans, peas, and lentils contain more protein than any other plant food, and they're also a good source of many vitamins and minerals that are commonly found in red meat, such as iron and B vitamins.

But that's where the similarities end, because as far as health is concerned, beans are a far wiser choice than red meat. For instance, unlike red meat, beans contain hardly any artery-clogging saturated fat. The fat they do contain is made up mostly of heart-healthy unsaturated fat. Another big difference is that legumes contain lots of cholesterol-lowering soluble fiber, whereas meat contains no fiber at all. At the same time, legumes are a good source of anticancer and heart-protecting phytochemicals, which, again, red meat contains none of.

If there is one draw back to replacing a red meat–based meal with a legume-based meal it is the question of protein. While the quality of protein in legumes is high, with the exception of soybeans, the quality isn't quite as high as the protein found in fish, shellfish, poultry, and meat. This is because legumes don't contain all the essential amino acids (the building blocks of protein) needed for growth and repair. Luckily this problem is easily overcome, because the amino acids missing from legumes are found in grain foods; and coincidentally, the amino acids missing from grain foods are found in legumes. So by mixing beans and grains together in one meal, you end up with a complete protein that is of the same quality as that found in fish, soybeans, and meat. Here are some good examples of legume and grain combinations that form a complete protein:

Baked beans on toast

Bean dip and baked corn chips

Bean risotto

Bean salad and crusty bread

Beans with pasta

Beans with rice

Chickpea stew served over couscous

Dahl (lentil curry) with rice or naan bread

Falafel kebab (gyro)

Hummus and pita bread

Lentil or bean burger

Lentil or bean soup served with bread

Tortilla bread with beans

The Fat-Fighting Powers of Legumes

One of the most visible benefits associated with adding more legumes to your diet is weight maintenance. Legumes are ideal for maintaining a healthy body weight for a number of reasons. First, they are only moderate in calories, which means you have to eat a great deal of them before they can do any damage. And it's very hard to eat too many legumes for the simple fact that they're bulky and high in fiber, which is nature's best appetite suppressant. Legumes are also effective for shedding those extra pounds because they contain natural carbohydrates, which give your body lots of energy to be more active—activity in turn burns body fat.

THE HEALTH-GIVING BENEFITS OF SOY

Although all legumes have health-giving properties, one legume stands out as being the healthiest of all—the soybean.

Soybeans have played an integral part in Asian culture, both as a food and as a medicine, for many centuries. In fact, according to ancient Japanese mythology, soybeans are a gift from the gods. And if recent scientific research is anything to go by, the humble soybean certainly lives up to this accolade.

SOY AND HEART DISEASE

Can soybeans reduce your risk of heart disease? If soy protein is substituted for meat protein the answer is yes, according to a report published in the *New England Journal of Medicine*. In the report, researchers at the University of Kentucky, Lexington, reviewed thirty-eight separate clinical studies on soy and found that people who substituted soy protein for about half of the meat protein in their diet reduced their LDL cholesterol by 12.9 percent and triglycerides by 10.5 percent. According to the lead author of the report, Dr. James Anderson, the results suggest that a diet that regularly includes soy has the potential to reduce heart-disease risk 25 to 30 percent.

SOY AND CANCER

Rates of breast and prostate cancer are low in Asia, where soy is eaten regularly. Scientists believe they have now identified one of the main reasons why soy could offer protection. Soybeans contain special phytochemical compounds called *isoflavones*. Research has shown that these compounds can work as powerful cancer blockers.

For example, the isoflavones in soy have been shown to block the growth of new capillaries that supply tumors with blood. Without an adequate blood supply, a tumor can't grow. Isoflavones have also been shown to directly inhibit the growth of different types of cancer cells in test-tube experiments.

And direct studies on soy consumption have shown just how powerful a cancer blocker it is. One study by researchers at Loma Linda University in California found that men who consumed soy milk at least once a day had a 70 percent lower risk of developing prostate cancer than those men who didn't. Another study by Dr. Wei Zheng of Vanderbilt University in Tennessee found that woman in China who consumed the most soy had the lowest risk of breast cancer.

SOY AND WOMEN'S HEALTH

Legumes in general have many health benefits for women, but studies have shown that soybeans in particular offer the most benefits. Part of the reason could be that soybeans contain high amounts of natural phytochemical compounds called phytoestrogens. These compounds are similar to the human hormone estrogen, except they are much weaker. As weak estrogens, these compounds act as a substitute form of estrogen in the body, and actually compete with the more potent estrogens made by a woman's body. As a result, phytoestrogens can help to regulate estrogen levels. This is of great importance to women because high estrogen levels have been associated with a range of problems, including increased risk of breast cancer, fibroid tumors of the uterus, and PMS.

The phytoestrogens found in soybeans are helpful not only when estrogen levels are high but when estrogen levels are low—such as during menopause—because they can provide much needed hormonal support for the body. This is why many of the symptoms of menopause that are taken for granted in the West, like hot flashes and night sweats, are rarely seen in countries where soy is a staple food. In Japan, for example, where soy products are consumed regularly, there isn't even a term for "hot flashes."

In addition, studies have shown that soybeans can slow down the loss of bone mass, which causes the bone-weakening disease osteoporosis.

THE MANY WAYS TO ENJOY SOY

Are you wondering how you can fit this remarkable protein-rich bean into your diet? Only a few short years ago the only soy products you were likely to see on the supermarket shelves were soy sauce and tofu. How times have changed! With all the media coverage that soybeans have received in recent years, Western consumers are demanding more soy products on their shelves—and these demands are certainly being met. These days the range of soy products available from your local supermarket is nothing short of remarkable. This is great news because now it's easier and tastier than ever to enjoy the benefits that soy has to offer.

Here are some tasty and nutritious ways that you can enjoy soy:

Dried soybeans. These can be used to replace any other variety of beans in dishes such as bean salad, homemade baked beans, or chili. The only drawback is that they take two to three hours to cook. Luckily you can now buy canned, precooked soybeans, which you can heat and eat in only minutes.

Fresh soybeans. Called *edamame* in Japanese, fresh soy is harvested while green and sold as "sweet beans" in Asian grocery stores in the summer months. Steamed or boiled in salted water, these make a great appetizer or snack, or they can be added to stir-fries.

Tofu (bean curd). Tofu is incredibly versatile because it has little taste of its own (but a delightful texture), which means that when you mix it with grains, vegetables, and seasonings, it soaks up their flavor. It comes in two main varieties: soft (silken) and firm. Firm tofu can be diced and sautéed in stir-fry dishes, and it can replace meat or poultry in casseroles, soups, and stews. Soft tofu can be used to replace soft cheese like ricotta in pasta dishes. It also adds creaminess to smoothies and when blended or puréed, it serves as a base for soups, sauces, dips, salad dressings, and desserts.

Baked, pressed tofu. This form of seasoned, extra-firm tofu comes in several marinade-type flavors and is ready to use straight off the supermarket shelf. Slice it and use it to replace meat as a tasty sandwich filling; serve it over noodles or rice, in salads, or with stir-fried vegetables.

Soy burgers. Soy burgers are a nutritious and delicious substitute for beef burgers. Serve them on a bun topped with fresh tomatoes, crisp lettuce, pickles, and your favorite sauce. There are lots of different varieties of soy burger patties, so experiment to find your favorite or try our version.

Soy hot dogs. We were amazed when we first ate a soy hot dog—it tasted just like the real thing (right down to that delicious smoky flavor). Treat them just like you would normal hot dogs and put them in a bun with all your favorite toppings.

Tempeh. This traditional Indonesian food is made from cooked and coagulated soybeans and is slightly higher in protein than tofu. It has a distinct flavor and a dense, chewy texture. Try it crumbled and used as a ground meat substitute; diced and sautéed, it can be tossed into rice, noodle, or vegetable dishes; and it can also be sliced and sautéed like cutlets and served with barbecue sauce.

Miso. Miso is a paste made from fermented soybeans, salt, and grains. It's delicious used as an all-purpose stock to flavor Asian dishes, casseroles, and soups. The only drawback is the high salt content, but this is offset somewhat by the fact that it is high in flavor, so you only need small amounts.

TVP (textured vegetable protein). Also known as textured soy protein (TSP), this versatile soy-based product can be used to replace ground beef in most recipes. It comes in dried form (so it keeps for extended periods), but when soaked in hot water for a short time it takes on the look and consistency of lean ground beef. Use it to partly or fully replace ground meat in dishes like burgers, tacos, sloppy joes, and spaghetti Bolognese.

Soy nuts. Soy nuts can be used in baked cakes, tossed into salads, or eaten by themselves as a snack.

Soy milk. Soy milk has come a long way since its early bland-tasting days and is now more than satisfactory as a replacement for regular milk. It's available at supermarkets in regular, low-fat, and flavored varieties such as chocolate, vanilla, and banana. Pour it over cereal, stir into hot drinks, or use in shakes, soups, or baking.

Soy bacon. I don't know how they do it, but soy bacon tastes and looks just like real bacon (it even has a white streak of "fat" on the side). Use soy bacon anywhere you would normally use bacon, such as in cooked breakfasts or sandwiches and salads.

Soy ham. Perfect diced in stir-fries, risottos, pasta dishes, and paellas or used cold as a sandwich filling. Soy ham also fries up nicely in a little oil and is perfect served with toast and eggs for breakfast.

NUTS AND SEEDS

Because of the high fat content of nuts, people in the West are often told to avoid them in order to reduce blood-cholesterol levels and prevent heart disease. But, as Dr. Frank Hu, a nutritional epidemiologist at Harvard School of Public Health points out: "In reality, nuts reduce your blood cholesterol and protect against heart disease because most of the fats in nuts are healthy fats—unsaturated fats, monounsaturated fats, polyunsaturated fats."

In fact, a study by Loma Linda University scientists in California on 34,000 people over six years found that those who consumed a handful of nuts four or more times a week had 50 percent fewer heart attacks than people who ate nuts less than once a week. A fourteen-year study at Harvard University involving more than 80,000 women showed similar results.

TYPES OF NUTS AND SEEDS

- Almonds
- Brazil nuts
- Cashews
- Chestnuts
- Linseeds (flaxseeds)
- Macadamia nuts

- Peanuts (actually a legume, not a nut, but it has the same nutritional profile as nuts and is used in the same way)
- Pecans
- Pine nuts
- Pistachios
- Sesame seeds
- Sunflower seeds
- Walnuts

Nuts and seeds aren't only a rich source of good fats, they also contain many other health-enhancing substances. For example, nuts and seeds are a good source of protein, fiber, vitamin E (a powerful antioxidant), magnesium, and zinc. Nuts also contain high amounts of an essential amino acid called arginine. This special protein has been shown to help relax blood vessels and make blood less sticky, which, in turn, reduces the risk of heart attack and stroke. And certain nuts and seeds—particularly walnuts, pecans, and linseeds (flaxseeds)—are a good source of omega-3 fatty acids.

The Perfect Snack Food

Snack foods are generally very high in fat. Most of this fat is hydrogenated vegetable oil, which contains high amounts of LDL-cholesterol-raising trans fat.

Nuts and seeds are other snacks that are high in fat; but most of the fat in nuts and seeds (except coconuts) is made up of heart-healthy unsaturated fats. But it's also important to remember that nuts are still high in calories. An ounce, which is about a handful, provides between 165 to 200 calories (depending on the type of nut). So the idea isn't simply to add nuts to your diet but to substitute them for other foods—especially less wholesome foods.

This works particularly effectively when you replace junk food with nuts, because calorie for calorie there is simply no comparison between the two. A donut, for example, is full of calories, but these calories come mostly from hydrogenated fat and sugar. So donuts contain very little in the way of nutrients and provide your body with no real sustenance. This means that not long after eating a donut, you'll be hungry again.

Nuts, on the other hand, are calorie rich but also nutrient rich. The fiber, protein, essential fats, and other nutrients in nuts sustain and nourish your body and satisfy your hunger for far longer than an equal number of calories from donuts or other "empty-calorie" snack foods ever could.

A Tasty Addition to Meals

As well as being a great snack food, nuts and seeds also make a delicious and healthy addition to meals. You can even use nuts to replace animal protein in a dish. Here are a few ways you can incorporate nuts and seeds into your meals:

- Adding a handful of cashews or slivered almonds to an Asian-style stir-fry, braise, or noodle dish makes a wonderful crunchy addition.

- Nuts go well with many pasta and risotto dishes. Pesto, for example, is a delicious sauce that comes from Genoa, Italy. It's made up of a mix of fresh basil, nuts (usually pine nuts), Parmesan cheese, garlic, and extra-virgin olive oil. It makes an incredibly delicious, creamy sauce that can be tossed through pasta or spread on bread or toast. Walnuts also make a rustic addition to pasta.

- Toasted sesame seeds sprinkled over a stir-fry add a wonderful flavor and texture.

- Crushed peanuts make a tasty and crunchy garnish for Thai, Indonesian, and Vietnamese dishes, and peanuts are one of the main ingredients in Indonesian satay sauce.

- Nuts add a flavor and texture boost to salads.

- Crushed nuts go perfectly sprinkled over cereal, oatmeal, yogurt, or fruit salad.

- Whole and crushed nuts and seeds can be added to your own homemade muesli.

- A handful of crushed almonds or pistachios is wonderful sprinkled over a Middle Eastern pilaf.

Drink and Be Merry

For thousands of years alcohol has occupied a prominent place in traditional Mediterranean and Asian cultures. The inclusion of moderate alcohol consumption in the Mediterranean and Asian pyramids reflects this fact. Researchers now believe that drinking alcohol daily, in moderation, isn't only an enjoyable social experience but can also benefit your body, particularly your heart and arteries.

LIQUID ASSETS

Does a drink a day keep heart attacks away? Yes, according to no fewer than sixty scientific studies that have shown alcohol to be protective against heart disease. Indeed, as far back as 1981 researchers from Johns Hopkins University School of Medicine, Baltimore, Maryland, cited more than a dozen studies in their article, "The Beneficial Side of Moderate Alcohol Use," which describes alcohol's heart-protective benefits. "A number of well designed and executed case-control studies," wrote Thomas Turner, MD, and colleagues in the *Johns Hopkins Medical Journal*, "indicate that the risk of coronary heart disease, especially myocardial infarction (heart attack), is lower in persons who use alcohol moderately than in abstainers."

In a scientific review published recently in the *British Medical Journal*, Harvard researchers looked at forty-two studies and concluded that regularly consuming alcohol in moderation equaled a 24.7 percent reduction in heart-disease risk.

WHICH ALCOHOLIC BEVERAGE
IS THE MOST HEART PROTECTIVE?

Research has found that *any* alcoholic drink (beer, wine, or spirits), when consumed in moderation, can raise your "good" HDL-cholesterol levels, thus helping inhibit the onset of heart disease. However, red wine has been found to contain other health-giving compounds that make it especially good for your health.

Unlike other alcoholic drinks, red wine is a rich source of a special group of phytochemicals called *phenolic compounds*, which are found in grape juice and particularly in grape skin. These compounds, which give grapes their color, have been shown to reduce the artery-clogging properties of LDL cholesterol, as well as to reduce the formation of blood clots and inhibit cancerous tumor growth. Phenolic compounds have a duel role, as they also work as powerful antioxidants, mopping up potentially dangerous free radicals that can destroy healthy cells, speed up the aging process, and increase your risk of heart disease and cancer.

This is why, out of all alcoholic beverages, red wine has been found to be the most protective. In one study, for example, Danish researchers followed more than 13,000 people over ten years and found that teetotalers had twice the risk of dying from heart disease as people who drank a moderate amount of red wine every day.

CONSUMING ALCOHOL WITH YOUR MEAL IS BEST

In the West, alcohol is often consumed before a meal or on its own. Throughout the Mediterranean and Asia, on the other hand, alcohol has traditionally been consumed at meal times. Recent research has shown that this interaction between food and alcohol could also help to explain some of the benefits associated with moderate alcohol consumption.

Dr. Maurizio Trevisan from the University of Buffalo, in New York, has reported—based on results from the Risk Factor and Life Expectancy (RIFLE) Study of more than 70,000 men and women in Italy—that benefits with respect to heart disease and overall mortality were more pronounced when wine was consumed with meals. His research helps support the results of a 1994 study by health researchers with the Japanese government that reported that wine with meals prevents the modification of LDL cholesterol to a form that can increase the risk of heart disease.

The consumption of alcohol at meal times also limits its abuse, according to Italian researcher Amedeo Cottino: "This is precisely what is meant by the very common Italian saying, 'Never drink wine between meals.' This ensures that alcoholic beverages never fill an empty stomach, and it also controls the amount of drinking by relating it to eating times."

HOW MUCH IS TOO MUCH?

Although alcohol certainly has its advantages, experts point out that there's only a small window of opportunity for deriving positive effects; this means that *modera-*

THE GREAT STRESS RELIEVER

The warm, relaxing feeling after one or two glasses of wine or beer goes a long way toward relieving the tensions of the day.

Dr. David Benton, a psychologist at the University of Wales, has been studying the impact of food and drink on behavior for over fifteen years and says that, in moderation, alcohol acts as a mild sedative. "In the short term, alcohol is a relaxant," he says. "It may even improve performance that has been disrupted by stress."

When combined with good food and conversation at the dinner table, the stress-relieving benefits of alcohol become even more pronounced. Unfortunately, the stress-relieving benefits of alcohol soon diminish when it's consumed in excess, and alcohol can end up working as a depressant. So take it easy and drink only in moderation—you'll get the best stress-relieving benefits that way.

tion is the key word. Studies have shown that around two drinks a day for men and one drink a day for women are the maximum limit (one drink equals 12 ounces of beer, 4 ounces of wine, 1.5 ounces of 80-proof spirits, or 1 ounce of 100-proof spirits). More than that and the advantages of alcohol start turning into disadvantages such as these:

Liver disease. If alcohol is consumed regularly in large amounts it can lead to a number of serious liver complaints such as cirrhosis of the liver, alcoholic hepatitis, and liver cancer.

Mouth and throat cancer. High levels of alcohol consumption increase the risk of cancers of the mouth, throat, and tongue.

Heart disease. Heavy drinkers are more susceptible to coronary heart disease and high blood pressure, and they are more likely to suffer a stroke.

Depression. A high level of alcohol intake can result in depression, memory loss, and mental deterioration.

Digestive disorders. Heavy drinkers may suffer from digestive tract diseases including gastritis, pancreatitis, and cancer of the upper digestive tract.

Another thing to remember is that alcohol is fairly high in calories, which means that if you consume too much alcohol you could easily gain weight.

Of course, it's important to note that these down sides only come about when you consume *too much* alcohol. If you follow the example of people from Mediterranean and Asian cultures and consume no more than one to two drinks a day, preferably with meals, then you only have to look forward to the benefits.

But, with that said, one of these days you'll no doubt find yourself in a situation where it's going to be difficult to have only a couple of drinks—for example at holiday celebrations or at a party. So what's the best solution? Well, you basically have two options:

- Find creative ways to consume less alcohol (more about this shortly) *or*

- Drink whatever is served and resume your healthy, moderate drinking habits immediately thereafter.

From a health point of view, you can choose option two without fear of ruining your well-being, as long as you limit this kind of activity to once in a blue moon. If you feel like taking option one by finding creative ways to consume less alcohol, here are some effective tips that you might find useful:

- Add some fresh fruit juice to champagne for a delicious champagne cocktail.

- Turn a glass of white wine into a spritzer by adding some soda water.

- Turn a glass of beer into a sweet refreshing shandy by adding some lemonade.

- Sip a nonalcoholic drink like a soft drink, cordial, soda, or mineral water (or just plain water) in between alcoholic drinks.

Remember that the first few drinks are usually used to quench your thirst. By quenching that thirst with a nonalcoholic drink first, you'll probably find you'll end up drinking less alcohol.

In short, consuming moderate amounts of alcohol (particularly red wine) is a simple and effective way to improve your health and relieve stress. The fact that it's also a highly pleasurable experience makes it all the more worthwhile. The cardinal rule is not to drink too much (no more than two drinks daily for men and one drink daily for women) and to make sure that you usually drink with your meal. If you follow these simple guidelines, you can feel confident in raising your glass and toasting to your health!

Stop Exercising, Start Living!

These days it almost seems as if there's a conspiracy to stop us moving. Most of us now have sedentary jobs that involve very little movement. Devices such as washing machines, vacuum cleaners, and dishwashers have reduced how much physical labor is required of us. Our leisure time revolves around passive activities such as watching TV, playing video games, or surfing the Internet. To top it off, our main form of transportation is now our car instead of our legs.

As a society we've virtually stopped moving. And when you don't move much, you dramatically reduce the number of calories your body burns. This, in turn, leads to weight gain. At the same time, lack of movement leads to a loss of muscle tissue. Muscles are active tissues that increase your fat-burning metabolism. In simple terms this means: the less muscle you have, the easier it is to get fat.

To make matters worse, by not moving much, your heart and other vital organs are not working as they should. This can increase the risk of heart disease, diabetes, high blood pressure, osteoporosis, and dozens of other potentially debilitating conditions. That's why movement is so important—every bit as important as eating the right foods.

The great news is that by moving your body only a little each day, it won't degenerate. You'll keep all your fat-fighting muscle tissue, your health and fitness will improve measurably, and you'll look and feel great. But when I say moving, I don't mean exercising. The fact is, the best way to bring movement into your life is to stop exercising and start living!

INCORPORATING PHYSICAL ACTIVITY INTO YOUR LIFE

The Mediterranean and Asian pyramids both include a reference to the importance of regular physical activity for maintaining good health. But the way Mediterranean and Asian peoples have gotten their physical activity for the past few thousand years hasn't been through exercising. When Professor Ancel Keys studied Greeks, Japanese, and Italians in the 1950s and '60s, he noted that most of them kept physically active by walking to see friends, gathering crops, pumping water, and carrying out other general day-to-day tasks. In fact, this is how humans have always kept physically active. We've never formally set aside time to exercise—not ever before in history. We just went about our day and, lo and behold, we stayed fit and in shape. These days, because modern technology has forced us into laziness, we think the only way to compensate is to set aside special time, put on special clothes, and formally "exercise."

What sorts of thoughts usually go through someone's mind when they're exercising? Most people aren't thinking, "Oh great, this is fun!" It's more likely to be "How much longer to go?" or "C'mon, I've got to keep this up for my own good." Ultimately, most of us are exercising not because we want to but because we think we have to.

But the simple fact is that we would all still be living in caves if our nature didn't dictate our need for diversity. Our senses crave stimulation to stay alert and engaged. For most of us, working out on the same exercise machine, jogging past the same sights, or just sticking to the same old exercise routine—no matter what it is—will eventually lead to boredom. And once boredom rears its head, it's only a matter of time before we give up altogether. Who can blame us!

NATURAL MOVEMENT

The revolutionary news is that you don't have to stick to a grueling structured exercise plan to get health benefits. The latest research reveals what history has always shown us: You can attain a good level of fitness simply by being more physically active in your everyday life.

The idea is to take the focus off formal "exercise" and put the emphasis on *natural movement*. By natural movement I simply mean moving as part of your everyday life— just like Mediterranean and Asian peoples have traditionally done for thousands of years. Of course, you can't be expected to start gathering crops or pumping water, but it doesn't matter, because there are lots of other ways you can slip movement unobtrusively into your hectic twenty-first-century lifestyle.

For example, instead of trying to find excuses not to exercise—like housework, shopping, and writing letters—why not make these tasks the regular exercise in your day? Think of everyday activities as an opportunity to kill two birds with one stone: in other words, accomplish a task and at the same time collect some movement.

Don't think of it as "having to do the housework," but instead use the chance to do a ten-minute aerobic workout by turning housework into a cardio-cleaning blitz. (You'll be amazed how vigorous vacuuming, dusting, and window cleaning can be!) Instead of circling to find a prime space, park at the far end of the lot and walk the rest of the way—adding another few minutes to your "activity bank." If you've got some shopping to do, use the opportunity to collect another five minutes and slip in a resistance workout by carrying your shopping bags to the car. And those letters you had to write—instead of mailing them by car on the way to use the treadmill at the gym, just walk to the mailbox instead (take the scenic route) and deposit another ten minutes into your activity bank so you can skip the gym altogether.

NO PAIN, ALL GAIN

Five minutes here, ten minutes there—without even thinking about it you've "exercised" for around half an hour today, just the right amount to enjoy the benefits that a healthy level of fitness offers. Before you know it, depositing movement into your activity bank will become as natural as brushing your teeth. After a few short weeks you'll notice improvements in your body tone and energy levels; you'll look better, get fitter, and generally feel great!

Our days are filled with activities that provide us with the chance to bring extra movement into our lives. Walking the dog (both you and your dog benefit), using the stairs (forget the Stairmaster!), and pushing the stroller or carriage (choose the hilly way for extra intensity) are all ideal activities you can do that happen to get you moving at the same time. Even the most unlikely times and places can provide the perfect opportunity to slip in some form of activity. For example, the bedroom can be very conducive to working up a light sweat. . . . I think you get the idea!

By using your imagination to slip activity unobtrusively into your busy lifestyle, you'll not only find you've exercised without even thinking about it, but you'll also have more time for yourself instead of spending it at the gym or fitness center.

Here are some other good examples of *natural movement*:

Clean your car by hand. Instead of taking your car through the gas station car wash, clean it at home by hand. Give it a good wash and polish with extra intensity. Washing your car by hand is also far gentler on your car's paintwork than taking it through a mechanical car wash.

Walk to your local store instead of driving. Walk to the local store for convenience items like milk and bread instead of taking the car or sending the kids. The physical benefits of brisk walking are many, including better endurance and an increase in your metabolic rate. Pop your small child in a shoulder carrier or push him or her in a stroller—the extra weight adds intensity and makes you work a little harder. Even subtle lifestyle changes like this are effective ways to add physical activity to your life and get you out into the fresh air and sunshine at the same time.

Park and walk. When you go to the mall, rather than circling the parking lot for the prime position closest to the entry, make a conscious decision to park as far away from the stores as possible and walk the extra distance instead. Although this may sound time-consuming, you'll probably find that you get inside the mall faster than if you circled around searching for a prime spot anyway.

Toil in the soil. Get out into the garden, get your hands dirty, and get your body moving. Mow the lawn, rake the leaves, weed the flower bed, dig holes, pot plants, and saw off overhanging tree limbs. All of these cardio-intensive activities contribute to the maintenance of your yard as well as your body. Although it's become commonplace for the time-poor, cash-rich among us to have a gardening service perform these tasks, why not experience the pride and satisfaction of doing them yourself? What's more, it's free and it can be fun!

Clean out your attic, basement, or garage. Spring-cleaning is a great way to get rid of all those boxes of unwanted stuff, as well as to help shed unwanted pounds. You'll be amazed at how active you'll get and astonished at how much junk you can clear in the process.

Walk to your local park for lunch. Instead of being stuck at home, at a desk, or in the office cafeteria, head to your local park or gardens instead. The fresh air is good for your lungs and the sunshine beats artificial lighting any day (vitamin D, which is essential for bone growth and maintenance, is also produced by the body when you're exposed to sunlight). A brisk walk and a change of scenery will do wonders for your physical and mental well-being. Even big cities have patches of green to use as a quiet respite from the hectic pace of modern life. Take off your shoes, loosen your tie, and close your eyes. Feed the birds with any leftover crumbs from lunch. Even after just a short time away, you'll return home or to work renewed and ready for the afternoon ahead.

Get to work on two wheels. Avoid traffic jams and cycle to and from work. Wear a helmet and have front and rear lights fitted to your bike if you plan to cycle at night. A word of caution: Long skirts and trouser cuffs tend to get caught in the bike chain, so wear more suitable clothing and change into your work clothes when you arrive—you'll be much fresher that way too!

Catch public transportation to work. Instead of driving to work, take the bus or train instead, which means walking to and from the bus stop or train station on both ends. Walking gives you a chance to plan the day ahead and arrive at work refreshed and alert. Likewise, a brisk walk after work gives you time to wind down and get some fresh air before arriving home. As well as the extra movement you're slipping into your life, you'll also save time and money (no more gasoline, parking fees, and traffic jams).

Shop and carry. One of the best ways to justify a shopping spree as a bona fide workout is to make a point of carrying your shopping bags on foot to the car or while you're window shopping. Just think—the more you buy, the better the workout! Similarly, cruise the supermarket aisles carrying a shopping basket instead of pushing a shopping cart around. The extra weight acts as resistance to give you an upper-body workout.

Park a few blocks from work. By walking the rest of the way, this burst of physical activity will give you a chance to stretch your legs and boost your metabolism before getting to the office. Alternatively, choose a parking space as far away from your building as possible and then walk the rest of the way at a brisk pace. Even the famous multimillionaire media mogul, William Randolph Hearst, had his limousine driver drop him off a few blocks from his mansion so he could walk the rest of the way home. It just goes to show that you're never too rich or too old to slip in some physical activity.

Work out at the office. If your job is sedentary and involves sitting at a desk in front of a computer screen for most of the day, use your initiative to incorporate movement in various ways. For instance, if you need to see colleagues on the fourth floor, take the stairs. Use the restroom that's most distant from your work area; if it's up several flights of stairs, great! Don't ask someone to bring you something, like a file or coffee; instead, go and get it yourself. Post the daily mail on foot rather than taking the company car. Walk to the local sandwich shop to get your lunch; if it's a block or two away, all the better. Instead of sending an interoffice memo or email, deliver it personally. These activities all add up to keep you more active and give you short, regular breaks in your work routine.

Walk and talk the kids to school. Rather than chauffeuring the kids to and from school, walk with them. Both you and the kids will benefit from the exercise, and it will give you the chance to have a good chat with them. Stop off on the way home from school at the playground or park and spend time with each other having fun. If your children catch public transportation, walk with them to and from the bus stop or train station instead of waving good-bye from the front door.

Make the most of vacations. Instead of using your vacation as an excuse to do nothing but eat too much and do as little as possible, use it as an opportunity to have fun and get moving at the same time. For instance, take a cycling tour through the countryside, go on a guided walking tour, go backpacking or mountaineering in national parks, or go kayaking or white-water rafting. Action-packed holidays are heaps of fun—see your travel agent for other ideas.

A LESSON IN NATURAL MOVEMENT

If you think it's going to be tough to add natural movement into your life because you're just "too busy," think again. Even people with the busiest lifestyles can still slip moderate physical activity into their everyday lives. A classic example is that of busy executive Geoffrey Cannon, director of science for the World Cancer Research Fund.

Cannon lives and works in busy central London, and in the 1990s he decided that it didn't make sense for him to own a car. He now mostly cycles to work, which takes around fifteen minutes each way. Sometimes, instead of cycling to work he walks twenty minutes to an underground station and at the other end he walks up the escalator (instead of just standing on it like a dead weight). He also doesn't use the elevator at work and walks up and down the stairs to see his work colleagues. As well, he regularly carries bags of food on foot or on his bicycle, and he walks to most of his appointments in central London.

This example clearly demonstrates that no matter how busy or hectic your life may be, there are always plenty of ways to slip in some natural movement.

FUN FITNESS

Slipping physical activity into your day-to-day tasks is a very effective way of getting lots of natural movement, but it certainly isn't the only way. Another good way of getting lots of natural movement is what Trudy and I call "fun fitness."

Helps control weight. In addition to burning calories while you're moving, physical activity also boosts your *basal metabolic rate*—the rate at which your body burns calories while at rest. In other words, when you're physically active, you continue to burn extra calories even after you stop moving.

Reduces the risk of heart disease. Heart disease is the Western world's leading cause of death. Physical activity helps prevent it by strengthening the heart, reducing blood pressure, lowering cholesterol, and combating obesity.

A study by researchers from the University of Washington in Seattle and the University of Michigan in Ann Arbor found that people who walk for exercise can reduce the risk of having a first heart attack by 73 percent and those who garden can reduce the risk by 66 percent compared with people who are not regularly physically active. "When performed for more than sixty minutes a week, walking for exercise or gardening was associated with a similar risk reduction to that of high-intensity leisure-time physical activity," reported Dr. Rozenn N. Lemaitre, who helped conduct the study.

Reduces high blood pressure and the risk of stroke. High blood pressure is a key risk factor for stroke, and regular physical activity has been shown to help reduce it.

Helps you live longer. Physical activity strengthens your heart and immune system and helps reduce the risk of atherosclerosis (clogged arteries), thus giving you a more robust age-fighting body. As Professor Ancel Keys noted while conducting the Seven Countries Study: "During the field work of this study it was not uncommon to see men [in Greece] of 80 to 100 years of age and more going off to work in the fields with a hoe."

Builds strength, flexibility, and stamina. When you move regularly your muscles become stronger, your joints become suppler, and you can remain active longer without tiring.

Helps preserve bone. Regular weight-bearing movement (walking, gardening, dancing, and the like) helps prevent the bone-thinning disease osteoporosis, which is a major health problem for many older women and men in the Western world.

Helps the body deal with stress. Regular movement strengthens your body's circulatory and immune systems. This in turn helps your body to better deal with the damaging effects of stress.

Improves love life. James White, PhD, director of the Human Performance Laboratory at the University of California in San Diego, recruited ninety-five healthy but sedentary men, average age forty-seven, into one of two exercise programs four days a week. One group engaged in low-intensity, sixty-minute walks. The other participated in an hour of aerobics. After nine months, both groups reported increased sexual desire and pleasure and more orgasms.

Improves sleep. When you move regularly throughout the day it helps your body wind down at night so you can sleep more deeply. This is why many sleep disorder experts recommend regular movement to treat insomnia.

As I mentioned earlier, exercising may keep your body active, but it usually fails to keep your mind active; more often than not, this means you eventually get bored and quit.

But what if an activity you do is fun and enjoyable, something that keeps your body and your mind active—surely you wouldn't be in such a hurry to give it up? For example, I love playing Frisbee. When I go out to play Frisbee, the last thing on my mind is exercising; I'm just having fun, doing an activity I enjoy. But without thinking about it I'm giving myself a full-body, cardio-intensive workout. Golf is another activity I enjoy doing that also happens to exercise my body at the same time. You can probably think of dozens of activities you enjoy that also happen to get you moving at the same time. To start you thinking, here are some more examples of *fun fitness*:

Go for a scenic walk. It's easy, free, and enjoyable. Let your mind roam freely and absorb the beauty of nature around you. For added enjoyment, buddy up with friends, family, and coworkers, or join a walking group. Depending on your level of fitness, you may want to walk fast for short distances or you may prefer to walk at a slightly slower pace for longer distances. Instead of walking the same way every time, explore different routes. Venture out into the countryside and hike along nature trails or go orienteering. Other good places to walk around include the zoos, art galleries, museums, and gardens.

Have a ball. Whether you opt for a football, soccer ball, baseball, softball, or basketball, throwing or kicking a ball around in your backyard or at the local park is great fun and provides excellent cardiovascular conditioning and coordination.

Dive in. Get fit in the water by heading to the local swimming pool for some aquatic activity. Most pools conduct classes such as aqua aerobics and swimming squads if you prefer a routine. But you don't need to join these structured programs to get the benefits of water exercise. If you get bored swimming up and down lanes, take a ball in with you and throw it around, or have a friendly game of water volleyball. As an added bonus, since water partially supports your weight and provides resistance to work against, gentle water exercises are excellent for people who suffer from back pain or other muscle or joint problems (including arthritis).

Go for a leisurely ride. Cycling is a great form of exercise, it's easy to fit into a busy schedule, and it's suitable for people of most ages and fitness levels.

Choose pleasant scenic routes and cycle ways that bypass heavily congested main roads or rush-hour traffic. For company, contact a local cycling club and join one of their regular riding tours. If you're the adventurous type, buy or rent a mountain bike, gear up with helmet and protective clothing, and head to the country.

Dance to the beat. Put on your favorite upbeat CD and have a dance around the house. If you have a partner, get him or her involved, or ask the kids to join in. Energetic dancing is a great way to condition your entire body. It uses all the major muscle groups and speeds up your metabolism. Who cares if you look a bit silly—unlike in a crowded aerobics class, no one is there to see you! If you're feeling social, why not head to a night club or dance club and enjoy a sweaty bop on the dance floor?

Go skating. Rollerblading and ice-skating help to build strong ankle and leg muscles and to develop balance. You'll get aerobic benefits if you push yourself hard and skate vigorously, using your arms to speed up, rather than gliding along with minimal effort. If you choose to skate outdoors, stay away from traffic and wear protective clothing. If the weather's inclement, head to the rink and, if you get bored skating around in circles, get involved in the games that are usually run.

Play with the kids. Encourage the kids to take a break from computer games for the old-fashioned excitement of real-life games in the open air: hide-and-seek, hopscotch, ball games in the yard, leapfrog, and jumping rope. All of these activities will get you and the kids outdoors for some physical activity and give you a chance to do something together.

Go to the beach. But don't just lie there like a beached whale. There are so many ways to give your body a fun seaside workout: go swimming or splash in the ocean, ride the waves on a surfboard, body board, or use your own body, play beach volleyball, fly a kite, paddle a kayak, or go sailing or windsurfing. Alternatively, enjoy more leisurely pursuits like building a sandcastle or walking along the beach.

Join a dance class. With so many dance styles available, you're sure to find one that appeals to you. Line, tap, belly, ballroom, rock 'n' roll, African, Latin, jazz—all are good for improving general fitness, flexibility, and well-being.

Dancing to music is a great way of improving your coordination, concentration, balance, memory, and rhythm, and it is a wonderful social activity. Don't worry if it's your first time; remember that everyone's a beginner at some stage, and there are usually classes especially designed with beginners in mind.

Go skiing. Whether you choose to ski on the snow (downhill or cross-country) or in the water (using skis or barefoot), skiing is an exhilarating activity that strengthens muscles and burns calories.

Try martial arts. Even if you're not interested in developing "fists of fury," martial arts can be a wonderful form of exercise for anyone to learn self-defense, gain confidence, and develop physical control. It's also a good outlet for stress. Apart from karate, there are many popular, less-demanding martial arts styles to choose from such as tai chi. Check your local telephone directory or the Internet to find a class that suits you, or learn at home from a book or video.

Play racquet sports. Tennis, badminton, squash, and table tennis are all fun ways to have an aerobic workout, build muscular strength and endurance, and improve balance and coordination. Book a tennis, squash, or racquetball court at your local sports center or buy your own gear and play at home. Even throwing a tennis ball against a brick or wooden wall is challenging and can be performed solo. Badminton sets (complete with net, racquets, and shuttlecocks) are cheap and can be set up in the backyard. Table tennis tables are relatively inexpensive new but are downright cheap purchased secondhand and can be folded up and wheeled away when not in use. Get family and friends involved in fun tournaments, or join local club fixtures if you're of a more competitive nature.

Fly a kite. Find a large open space (such as a park or beach) and return to your childhood by flying a kite. Not only does flying a kite involve plenty of physical activity, but it also improves your hand-eye coordination.

COMPETITIVE SPORTS

It's amazing what a bit of friendly competition can do to up your fitness without you even thinking about it. Competitive sports (where you're playing against someone else) is one of the easiest ways to have a high-intensity workout without pain—in fact, quite the opposite. You're focused on the match, you're having fun and enjoying yourself, yet at the same time you're getting fit and healthy. Competitive sports like basketball, softball, baseball, or football are also good for relieving stress and are great for making new friends and expanding your social life.

The benefits of incorporating more activity into your life are overwhelming: a leaner body, more energy, less disease, and a longer life. And fitting physical activity into your life, as you've discovered, is a pretty straightforward affair. As a bonus, you no longer have to put yourself through sweaty workouts or boring, structured exercise routines in order to get fit. The key now is simply to incorporate some form of physical activity into your life on a regular basis. The rewards will speak for themselves.

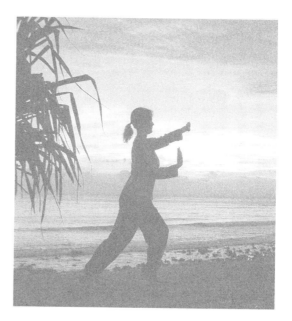

A Healthy Mind
in a Healthy Body

Achieving optimal health isn't just about looking good on the outside—it's also about feeling good on the inside. This has been known for thousands of years throughout Asia and the Mediterranean region, and the ancient Romans even had a saying for it: *mens sana in corpore sana*, which literally means "a healthy mind in a healthy body."

Although there are many effective ways that you can go about improving your physical health, exactly what steps can you take to directly improve your emotional health?

Learning from the traditional cultures of the Mediterranean region and Asia, as well as from our own personal experiences, we believe there are five fundamental ways that you can substantially improve your emotional health and well-being:

1. Enjoy good food and the rituals surrounding it.

2. Have a more relaxed and optimistic attitude toward life.

3. Truly appreciate the people and things around you.

4. Pursue your passions.

5. Set aside "calm time" each day.

Let's take a look at each of these steps in detail, starting with one of my favorite subjects: food!

ENJOY GOOD FOOD AND
THE RITUALS SURROUNDING IT

There can be no doubt that the food you'll be eating as part of a MediterrAsian way of living is very good for your body in a physical sense. But so far we haven't touched much on the emotional aspect of food.

Food is not simply fuel, as some would like us to believe. Food is one of life's wonderful and glorious pleasures. Good food uplifts the emotions; provides comfort, satisfaction, and a sense of well-being; and can be spiritually fulfilling.

Think of all the senses that are involved when you enjoy good food: the smell, the sight, the texture, and the taste. You're smelling, seeing, feeling, as well as tasting—talk about hitting a lot of senses at the same time. Is it any wonder we love food so much?

Unfortunately, although the enjoyment of food should be one of the emotional highlights of our lives, in Western society good-tasting food is usually associated with food that's bad for you. This is very often true.

Many popular Western foods that taste good also happen to be loaded with calories, and at the same time they fall short in the nutrient department. Because of this, many of us have come to associate good-tasting food with food that's unhealthy and fattening.

But good-tasting food and food that's good for you certainly don't have to be mutually exclusive. Far from being unhealthy and fattening, traditional Mediterranean- and Asian-style foods taste delicious, but they're typically packed with nutrients and contain only a moderate number of calories. This means that this food satisfies the stomach, the senses, and the soul—all without compromising your health.

The Emotional Pleasures of Food

So, by eating the MediterrAsian way, you can start rejoicing over food, savoring it, getting full and satisfied—all without guilt. This is how people from the Mediterranean region and Asia have done it for centuries. They've always eaten lots of good-tasting food that made them feel good—physically *and* emotionally.

Indeed, the emotional aspect of food has always been a point to be celebrated in Mediterranean and Asian cultures. Traditionally, mealtimes have been cherished and enjoyment of the food seen as paramount. In Italy, for example, they use the term *"Mangia!"*—which means "eat!" But according to Italian-American food writer Anthony Del Plato, it means much more than that. To Italians, *mangia* means "eat and enjoy this food, relish all food, taste as much as you can, eat up life, eat and be well!"

This same fundamental philosophy is shared throughout the Mediterranean region and equally in Asia, where enjoyment of food has always been regarded as a deep-rooted part of the emotions and mealtimes are considered a blissful ritual.

More Than Just Food

The emotional fulfillment that eating provides doesn't just come from the enjoyment of the food—your surroundings can often be equally important.

In the Mediterranean region and in Asia, mealtimes are traditionally seen not only as a time for eating wonderful food but also as a time for relaxing, de-stressing, coming together with friends and family, and enjoying good conversation and a good laugh.

From our own personal experience, we have certainly found that sharing the pleasure of good food washed down with wine or cold beer is very conducive to relaxation, conversation, and laughter! And because of this, mealtimes (particularly dinnertime) have become one of the most emotionally and spiritually fulfilling times of the day for us.

We've also discovered something else quite extraordinary—the preparation and cooking of MediterrAsian-style meals can be a very fulfilling experience in its own right.

Unlike a typical Western meal, where the most exotic flavorings are usually salt, pepper, and ketchup, Mediterranean and Asian dishes contain a host of wonderful fragrant herbs, spices, and condiments. And instead of bland, colorless, lifeless ingredients to work with, there are lots of vegetables, fruits, fish, beans, nuts, and grains—in all sorts of shapes, colors, sizes, and textures. It's a true pleasure for the senses preparing and cooking these sorts of ingredients. And we still constantly marvel at how such simple ingredients can be transformed so quickly into such wonderful creations.

We also find that the time we spend in the kitchen preparing and cooking is a great bonding experience. Coming together and working to achieve something is a great way to catch up and get in touch with each other. And it really gives us a tremendous sense of achievement when we sit down to enjoy the meal knowing that it was created from the fruits of our own labor.

Of course, although we get a lot of emotional satisfaction from preparing and cooking meals at home, it certainly doesn't stop us from regularly eating out at Mediterranean- and Asian-style restaurants. Greek, Italian, Chinese, Spanish, Japanese, Indian, Moroccan, Lebanese, Thai, and Vietnamese restaurants are some of our favorites.

Because these types of restaurants have a large number of dishes that fit within MediterrAsian eating guidelines, we get the emotional satisfaction of enjoying good-tasting food that's good for us, with the added bonus that we don't have to clean up afterward!

Eat to Your Heart's Content

Food is *not* a science experiment. It isn't something that should be counted, weighed, and dissected—it should be savored and thoroughly enjoyed. And by eating the

MediterrAsian way, you really can enjoy the pleasures of eating to your heart's content—your emotional heart as well as your physical heart.

HAVE A MORE RELAXED
AND OPTIMISTIC ATTITUDE TOWARD LIFE

Enjoying lots of delicious food throughout the day is great for improving your emotional well-being; but there's a lot more to life than just mealtimes. So how do you go about looking after your emotional well-being at other times of the day?

Again, we can learn a great deal from the traditional cultures of the Mediterranean region and Asia. A common trait throughout these cultures is that people generally have a more relaxed and laid-back attitude to life. Simple celebrations of daily life are also common. And there's a general acceptance that life is fleeting and that time, as well as loved ones and friends, are precious commodities that can't be taken for granted.

We believe that having a similar attitude in your own life is one of the key steps to dramatically improving your emotional well-being. But in this chaotic, high-stress twenty-first-century Western world, how can you possibly have the same laid-back, optimistic attitude to life as people from traditional Mediterranean and Asian cultures?

Well, there's no doubt that the twenty-first-century Western world can be a highly stressful environment to live in—stressful events seem to bombard us constantly. And this constant stress doesn't affect just our emotional health and well-being—it can also have a direct impact on our physical health (see the sidebar "The Stress Story," page 83). But it's very important to remember one simple point: your *attitude* determines your stress level.

Stress and Perception

You may have noticed that some people are virtually immune to stress. No matter what comes up, they seem to be able to deal with it, often without batting an eyelid. Could it just be a case of enormous self-control? Perhaps. But part of the reason could lie in the fact that each of us has a different perception of what is stressful.

More than two thousand years ago the Greek philosopher Epictetus said that it's never the things that happen to us that upset us, it's our view of these things. In other words, it's *your* view of an event that makes it stressful and not the event itself.

As an example, in 1900, the polar explorer Sir Ernest Shackleton put the following advertisement in the *London Times*:

Men wanted for hazardous journey. Small wages, bitter cold, long months of complete darkness, constant danger, safe return doubtful. Honor and recognition in case of success.

You wouldn't really expect many people, if any, to reply to such an advertisement. But, surprisingly, there were hundreds of eager responses. This shows that what some people may find stressful, others may find desirable.

As another example, you've probably noticed that when some people get caught in a traffic jam they soon become frustrated and "stressed-out" and often shout at the cars ahead or pound on the horn. Yet, at the same time, other people who are caught in the same traffic jam are quite calm. In the end, it's the same situation, but it leads to two completely different reactions.

Both of these examples demonstrate that stress is an emotional state—it's not the situation itself but your view of the situation that makes it stressful. Unfortunately, the stress that starts in your mind can end up affecting your emotions, your body, and your spirit (see "The Stress Story").

HOW TO CHANGE YOUR VIEW OF A STRESSFUL SITUATION

Inside each of us we have the power to control whether a situation becomes stressful or not. What it basically comes down to is changing your mindset when a situation arises that you would usually find stressful—for example, accidentally backing into the neighbor's fence, having a stack of bills all arrive at the same time, trying to meet an important deadline, or having your car break down, and so on.

Instead of seeing these events as stressful, change your perception and look at these events from a more optimistic viewpoint. And I don't mean "head in the clouds" optimistic; I'm talking about being a realistic optimist. Being a realistic optimist means that you're aware that life is inevitably going to throw you curveballs, but instead of see-ing these curveballs as *problems*, you see them as *challenges*.

After my accident I spent a fair amount of time wallowing in self-pity, and it just got me more and more stressed and depressed. But when I changed my mindset and saw a challenge instead of a problem, it was like a switch had gone off in my head. It immediately made everything much easier to deal with, and I felt a lot happier and much more in control. This experience showed me that emotional pain can often be worse than physical pain—but at the same time I also learned firsthand that emotional pain really is self-induced.

These days, when a situation arises in my life that could be stressful, I like to ask myself this simple question: *"Is getting worried about it going to help or hinder the situation?"* I soon realize that no matter what the problem is, worrying about it certainly won't help—but turning it into a challenge will. In other words, instead of crying over spilled milk, I just clean it up and get on with my life.

There's nothing new about stress, nor is it an unnatural phenomenon. Stress is actually a kind of ancient survival mechanism built into us by thousands of years of evolution. When our pre-historic ancestors were confronted with danger (like a hungry saber-toothed tiger), this set off an instant survival reaction that caused changes in body chemistry, including increased heart rate, higher blood pressure, and a release of large amounts of the hormone adrenaline—all in preparation for either a physical showdown or a hasty retreat! After this "fight or flight" reaction, the body would return to its normal, relaxed state. This biochemical reaction to external pressure is popularly known as stress.

Although stress is nothing new, the amount of stress we're now dealing with on a day-to-day basis is higher than ever before. These days we're constantly subjecting our stone-age bodies to space-age lifestyles—from traffic jams and noisy, crowded cities to juggling responsibilities and family arguments—all combined with our ongoing struggle to balance work, relationships, children, and finances.

The Dangers of Stress

What happens when we're constantly in a state of high stress? Instead of returning to the desirable, relaxed post-stress phase, the body adapts to the pressures, so in effect your body ends up being in a constant state of fight or flight. Constricted blood vessels, increased heart rate, and high blood pressure become permanent fixtures. Under these circumstances, we begin to measurably harm our health.

In the end, too much stress can lead to a range of problems, including neck, shoulder, and back pain; frequent headaches; attacks of arthritis and asthma; and bowel irregularities and digestive problems. High levels of stress have also been identified as a key risk factor for heart disease and stroke.

So, what's the best way to deal with all this unhealthy stress? Should you pack up all your belongings and move into the nearest cave or become a monk and meditate all day? Far from it! By following the simple guidelines outlined in this chapter, you'll be well on the way to sub-stantially lowering your stress levels.

Obviously, all situations aren't going to be so easy to deal with, but always remember that no matter what the situation is, worrying about it definitely won't help—*it will only make it worse.*

In the end, you're the one in control, and it is you who determines how you deal with any situation that arises in your life. However, by having a more optimistic attitude and seeing challenges instead of problems, you will find it much easier not only to deal with stress but not to let a situation turn stressful in the first place.

Having a positive outlook on life and turning life's curveballs into challenges may seem like a relatively straightforward thing to accomplish with life's minor ups and downs. But what about really major, life-changing events like the death of a loved one, losing your job, going through a divorce, or a major accident?

How is it possible in these circumstances simply to look for positives and turn these events into challenges? Actually, in exceptional circumstances like these it's more important than ever to have an optimistic outlook.

I think someone who epitomizes seeing the positives in the worst of situations is Alex Zanardi, a champion Italian race car driver who found fame when he won the prestigious and grueling CART (Championship Auto Racing Teams) motor-racing series back-to-back in 1997 and 1998. But Zanardi's outstanding career was abruptly cut short during the 2001 CART World Series. While leading the race at the American Memorial 500 in Lausitz, Germany, Zanardi pulled in to make a routine pit stop with thirteen laps to go. As he exited the pits, his car skidded, he lost control, and the car veered across the track into the path of a race car traveling at almost 200 miles an hour.

The horrific accident tore Zanardi's car in half and sprayed debris across the track. He was quickly rushed by helicopter to a Berlin hospital; but due to the severity of Zanardi's injuries, doctors had to amputate both his legs above the knee.

Despite losing both his legs, the medical staff was amazed by Zanardi's quick recovery, as well as his mental resilience. In fact, less than a month after the accident Zanardi was conducting interviews with the media from his hospital bed. In one interview with the *Associated Press* he said in a strong and cheerful voice, "I can't complain. I'm in good condition. . . . I lost my legs, but my upper body is strong, my energy is back and I move around with my arms and I'm pretty independent about everything."

Although he was highly optimistic, Zanardi was also realistic about his circumstances. In an interview with the Italian magazine *Autosprint* he said, "I'm trying to get through this in the most positive way possible. I don't think about what I lost, but everything I've still got, which I've realized is a great deal. . . . I've always looked forward and that's what I intend doing this time. There have been difficult moments and I know there will be more in the future, but with every day that goes by things are getting better. Even my legs, what's left of them, I'm learning to control my movements better. I want to, and I must, think positively. I've got a new life ahead of me and now I want to use all my energy to make the most of it."

Even though it looked like Zanardi's racing career was over, in 2003 Zanardi stunned everybody by reappearing at the same racetrack where he had nearly lost his life in 2001. Aided by a hand-operated brake and accelerator, he symbolically drove the thirteen laps he wasn't able to complete when he had last been on the track.

Later that year he drove a specially modified sports car at Monza in his first full race since the accident. Zanardi not only finished the race, but, after starting near the back of the field, he placed a competitive seventh. Amazingly, in 2004, Zanardi completed a full season, and now he's back racing full-time again after being signed by BMW.

Alex Zanardi's typically positive Mediterranean attitude toward adversity is a lesson for all of us when we go through rough patches in life. No matter how dire a situation may seem, having a positive, optimistic attitude and seeing a challenge instead of a problem will always be the best way of getting through it.

The Longevity Bonus

Having a more optimistic outlook toward life's ups and downs doesn't just benefit you now by reducing your stress levels; it can also benefit you in the future by increasing your life span. Scientists have long suspected that an optimistic outlook can help people live longer, and now two recent studies have confirmed just that.

One study of 160 centenarians (people who live to 100 and older) living in Boston found that most of them tended to have a similar mindset. According to Margery Silver, EdD, a neuropsychologist at Harvard Medical School and associate director of the study: "They are usually positive, optimistic people, who handle stress extremely well. They also tend to be resourceful and adaptable. There are people in our study who survived the Holocaust and others who went through other terrible hardships. They just were able to adapt to their situation, maintaining a positive attitude. When they have a problem or setback, they figure out a way to deal with it."

Another study, by researchers at the Mayo Clinic in Minnesota, also found that people with a more optimistic view on life tended to have longer life spans. In the study, researchers compared results from a personality test taken by participants thirty years earlier with their subsequent mortality rates. It was found that those who scored high on optimism had almost 20 percent less risk of premature death than did those who scored high on pessimism.

"It confirmed our commonsense belief," reported Toshihiko Maruta, MD, a psychiatrist at the Mayo Clinic and lead author of the study, "it tells us that mind and body are linked and that attitude has an impact on the final outcome—death."

TRULY APPRECIATE THE PEOPLE AND THINGS AROUND YOU

Of course, it's always going to be a lot easier to be optimistic about life's up and downs when you have a positive frame of mind to begin with. But you can't simply force yourself into having a positive frame of mind; it's something that has to be developed naturally. But *how*?

From our own personal experience, we have found that a good way to start naturally developing a positive frame of mind is by not taking things for granted in life. It's a sad fact that many of us are so caught up in the routine of our day-to-day lives that we often neglect to truly appreciate life and those around us. We forget how important things are to us, and it's usually only after they're gone that we truly appreciate how much they're really worth to us.

I've often read about people who've been diagnosed with terminal cancer and how suddenly they get a new appreciation of life and the things around them. Many of these people even say that, although they may be dying, they are actually "living" more than they ever have before.

By this, they mean they are seeing the world from a different perspective. Nothing can be taken for granted anymore, and even things that most of us would think of as trivial, such as the feeling of wind through your hair or the warmth of sun on your face, become much more important and special.

Stop and Smell the Roses

It doesn't have to take a terminal illness to heighten your appreciation of the people and the things around you. It's all about having the realization in your own life that time in this world, for all of us, really is quite fleeting—but rejoicing in this fact and seeing time as the precious commodity that it is. It's about realizing that once a day of your life is gone you can never have it back again, and thus making the most of it and appreciating all the wonderful things around you in life: the company of friends and loved ones, the taste and texture of good food, the smell of freshly baked bread, the storekeeper's smile, the sounds of children playing, the colorful marvels of nature, the fact that all your trillions of cells are working in remarkable harmony to keep you alive.

Having genuine gratitude for life and those around you truly enriches your spirit and makes life much more emotionally fulfilling. And, as a natural consequence, it's also a great way of creating a much more positive frame of mind.

PURSUE YOUR PASSIONS

Along with being grateful, another very important way you can develop a naturally positive frame of mind is by pursuing the things in life you feel truly passionate about. It's easy in life to sometimes feel like you're adrift on a huge ocean with no compass; but having a passion helps give you direction and brings more meaning to your life. To identify what your true passions are in life, simply follow your heart and really explore what fulfills and excites you.

You might have a passion for writing, cooking, decorating, animals, computers, helping others, sport, mathematics, teaching, crafts, music, or like me, your passion could be art. Whatever your passions are, be proactive and pursue them with vigor. And if you can find a way to turn your passion into your job, then you'll never have to "work" another day in your life.

That's exactly what my stepfather, Lindsay, did. When he was in his forties, he felt "stressed out" and stuck in a rut, working as a sales manager. However, one of the things he was really passionate about in life was home brewing. He would spend hours at a time out in the backyard shed brewing and bottling beer—and he *loved* every minute of it.

So he decided to quit his job, combine his sales experience with his passion for home brewing, and start his own home brew shop. He now owns and runs his own successful home-brewing shop, and, needless to say, he feels much more fulfilled and positive about life.

SET ASIDE "CALM TIME" EACH DAY

Enjoying good food and the rituals surrounding it, having a more optimistic attitude toward life, truly appreciating the people and things around you, and pursuing the things in life you are passionate about are all great ways of reducing stress and improving your emotional and spiritual well-being

But there is one other *very important* way you can substantially improve your emotional and spiritual well-being. We call it "calm time." Simply put, calm time is a special time just for you (or you can share it with someone close). It's a time to relax, rejuvenate, and reconnect with your spirit.

The Principle of Calm Time

Just as you need to sleep each day to be physically recharged, you also need time each day to de-stress and to recharge your emotional and spiritual energy.

For centuries Mediterranean and Asian people have made a point of setting aside special time to relax and rejuvenate their minds and bodies. The afternoon siesta in Italy, Spain, and Greece and meditation, yoga, and tai chi in Asia are good examples of such time. But calm time can also be as simple as sitting in the garden admiring the beauty of nature or relaxing in a hot bubble bath with candles and incense burning. As long as it's relaxing and enjoyable—it's *calm time*.

Trudy and I always make sure we set aside at least thirty minutes for calm time each day (not necessarily in one block of thirty minutes). We realize that this time of emotional and spiritual rejuvenation is just as important for our overall health and well-being as what we eat and how much we move.

Over the years we've discovered there are dozens of fun and enjoyable ways to relax, rejuvenate, and reconnect with our spirit—and we're sure you'll have no trouble regularly incorporating some of these ideas into your own life.

Soak in a hot bubble bath by candlelight. Shed your clothes and daily concerns and relax in a good old-fashioned hot bath, full to the brim with creamy bubbles. Let all your tensions evaporate with the dissolving foam. Make sure your favorite music is playing in the background. And don't forget to accompany those burning candles with a stick or two of incense. If you don't have a bathtub, have a long relaxing soak under a hot shower instead.

See a funny film. Go to the cinema or rent a comedy movie on video or DVD and laugh until you cry. Laughter is one of the healthiest antidotes to stress. When you laugh, or even just smile, blood flow to the brain is increased, endorphins (painkilling hormones that give you a sense of well-being) are released, and levels of stress hormones drop. And, besides, life's too serious—so laugh as long, loud, and often as you can.

Surf the Web. There are literally millions of words, pictures, sounds, videos, and animations out there in cyberspace. And, for just a few dollars each month, you can have unlimited access to it all (as long as you have a computer or similar device, of course). Everything from thousands of Mediterranean and Asian recipes to the latest Hollywood gossip is at your fingertips.

Keep a diary or journal. Writing down your feelings in a diary or journal can help you get in touch with your soul as well as relieve emotional stress. In a study conducted by psychologist James W. Pennebaker, PhD, from Southern Methodist University, in Texas, participants wrote for twenty minutes a day over four consecutive days about issues or emotions that were causing them stress. When the study was completed, participants showed improved mental health and were better able to cope with stress.

Relax in the garden. Set up that old hammock, throw down a comfy rug, or just lounge on a patch of grass and soak up the sunshine (don't forget the sunscreen!). If you like to rejuvenate but also want to get more than a sunbath, why not get in touch with Mother Nature and get your hands dirty by tending to an herb garden or planting a tree? The garden is a wonderful sanctuary that is ideal for both mindless leisure activities and more practical pursuits. If your own garden is little more than a couple of pots on the window ledge, then head to a public park or garden nearby for some regular botanical therapy.

Visit parks, gardens, and nurseries. Stop and smell the flowers, play on the swings (you're never too old), or throw a Frisbee or ball around. Instead of heading straight to the office cafeteria at break time, relax by yourself or with a friend at the nearest park and take in the fresh air and scenery. Even the local plant nursery is a wonderful place to immerse yourself in the natural beauty of the plant kingdom—and you can even take a little piece home with you.

Have a massage. Enjoy a relaxing massage from the tips of your toes to the top of your scalp—wherever tickles your fancy. Call your local salon for a rundown of their services and the types of massage offered including Swedish, reflexology, or Reiki. Or exchange favors with your partner and give each other a gentle massage with a little oil and lots of TLC. The soothing experience will give you a chance to revive sore muscles and leave your entire body feeling renewed.

Read or write poetry. Read works by your favorite poet. Make sure you find a relaxed room away from noise, and totally absorb yourself in the words as they unravel from the page. Or go a step further and write your own poetry.

Get a new hairstyle. Is it time for a change? If you're on the way to a new body, then why not go the whole hog and change your hair at the same time? If you've always had long hair, why not go short? Try highlights, or even go radical and change your hair color completely. The possibilities are endless, and one thing's for sure—you'll have plenty of fun in the process!

Paint or draw a picture. Grab some crayons, pencils, oils, pastels, or ink and express yourself on paper, canvas, or paint digitally on a computer. If you think you're lacking in natural artistic ability, think about joining an art class. For inspiration, get art books from the library or bookstore, or visit your local art gallery.

Learn to play an instrument. Either take lessons or grab some sheet music and teach yourself at your own pace. If you used to play music in a school band, reacquaint yourself with your old instrument. Or maybe there's a closet rock star hidden somewhere . . . why not find out?

Learn another language. Learning to speak and write another language is a great way of increasing your life skills, and it's also a relaxing experience. Find a language that appeals to you on an emotional level and learn the language by yourself, or get your partner involved and learn together.

Plan your next holiday escape. Pick up a few holiday brochures at your local travel agent for some getaway ideas. Be adventurous and plan a trip to exotic, faraway places or maybe just a fun weekend away somewhere closer to home.

Watch a classic movie. Sink back in your sofa, dim the lights, and travel back to another time and place courtesy of the classic video or DVD of your choice. Some of our favorites include *Wuthering Heights* (1939), *Rear Window* (1954), *It's a Wonderful Life* (1946), *Rebecca* (1940), *The Adventures of Robin Hood* (1938), *It Happened One Night* (1934), and *Some Like it Hot* (1959).

Visit the library. Take some time out and browse through the shelves for books and magazines that interest you. Read in the peace and quiet of the library or borrow some books to read at home.

Chat on the Internet. Hook up to the Internet, and you can talk (well, type actually) to people from all over the world for the price of a local call. People "chat" about thousands of different topics, among them health, fitness, and recipes. If you don't have Internet access at home, book an hour or two at an Internet café. Most libraries also have Internet facilities for public use.

Look through old photos and home movies. Dust off your old photos, or dig out your home movies. Get nostalgic and reminisce about old memories from your past (only good ones, of course!).

Go for a sightseeing drive. With a local map or street directory in hand, go exploring in your car. Most towns and cities have pleasant areas for a leisurely drive on a Sunday afternoon. Check out the local scenery, sights, and sounds and discover places that you've never been before.

Treat yourself to some aromatherapy. Drop some essential oil in an oil burner or put a few drops in a running bath, and let the fragrances invigorate you.

Go to the zoo. Marvel at the animal kingdom firsthand. Watch the frenzy of animals at feeding time and take the opportunity to feed the animals. If there's no zoo in your area, find an animal sanctuary or reserve, feed some ducks or squirrels in the park, or just take a moment to watch any local native wildlife, including birds.

Play a fun leisure game. Darts, pool, table tennis, and bowling are always favorites.

Take up pottery. If you've ever seen the movie *Ghost* you'll appreciate that pottery can be a whole lot of fun. There's nothing quite like the feeling of slippery, wet clay oozing through your fingers. This stress relief alone makes pottery a worthwhile experience. The fact you can create your own pots, plates, vases, and cups is an added bonus!

Rent or buy some fun and entertaining software. Check out the latest cookbook or encyclopedia on CD or DVD, or try your hand at one of the latest 3D games.

Make love. Set aside a special time to relax and share intimacy with the one you love. Create the right mood with soft lighting, music, and perfume. Share your fantasies and experiment with different positions, locations, and times.

Take photos. It's a relaxing experience to enjoy pleasant surrounds and forever be able to capture the moment on film. Why not start up special albums and fill them full of different shots (for example, a nature album or a baby album)?

Get a pet. Whether it's a dog, cat, bird, or fish, a pet can play a vital role in stress relief. Pets can also be good for your heart. A Johns Hopkins Medical

Center study found that fifty out of fifty-three people with pets were alive a year after their first heart attacks, while only seventeen of thirty-nine of those without pets lived a year.

Visit a museum or local art gallery. Walk among the exhibits and explore in detail the ones that interest you.

Play a board game. Monopoly®, chess, Trivial Pursuit®, checkers, and Scrabble® are some good examples.

Do a crossword puzzle. Completing a crossword not only enhances your knowledge of words, but it's also a great way of relaxing and de-stressing.

Play a game of cards. Try your hand at solitaire or get together with friends for a game of poker or gin rummy.

Meditate. Meditation is a quick and relaxing way to take your mind away from troubling and stressful thoughts. Go deep within yourself or just catch a few quiet moments in the solitude of a private room. Choose somewhere you are relaxed and happy and simply "chill out." For information on different meditation techniques, purchase a book on the subject or research under "meditation" and "breathing techniques" on the Internet.

Book into a day spa. Day spas provide a little bit of luxury for everyone. Try one of the beauty treatments and other self-indulging services that are offered.

Chill out at the beach. Listen to the sounds of the ocean, drench yourself in the refreshing surf, or just read your favorite novel on the warm sand.

Write a letter or e-mail. Whether you want to catch up with an old friend or find out the latest family gossip, take the time to share your news in a letter. For something more immediate than snail mail, why not e-mail your thoughts instead? You can send your message from home if you have Internet access, or stop by an Internet cafe or library to "post" your e-mail.

Phone friends, family, or a lover. Have a good old gossip with a friend or family member. Or maybe a long and personal chat with someone more intimate.

Listen to your favorite music. Select a CD to suit your mood. Give yourself a chance to put your feet up, then sit back, close your eyes, and be taken away by the music, lyrics, and memories.

Read a book or magazine. What are you in the mood for—a thriller, a romance, or maybe a mystery? Or perhaps a nonfiction title or glossy magazine is more your style. Find somewhere relaxed and quiet (snuggled in bed is always a good option), and read it cover to cover.

Soak your feet. Give your feet a treat and fill a bowl with warm water and a few drops of aromatherapy oil of your choice. Let the warm water soothe away the day's tensions and leave your feet supersoft.

Relax in front of an open fireplace. Watch the burning logs, listen to the crackling flames, and allow the warmth to penetrate your inner being.

Practice tai chi. Tai chi is practiced by millions of Chinese and Japanese every day, and in recent years this ancient martial art has become increasingly popular in the West. The slow, controlled, dancelike movements of tai chi can be helpful in achieving a state of total relaxation of the whole body, which helps to quiet the mind and promote relaxation. A study in China observed a group of 120 people between 50 and 80 years of age who had practiced tai chi for many years. They found that after practice, 92 percent of the group became noticeably more cheerful and optimistic.

Practice yoga. Yoga originated in India more than three thousand years ago. Although there are several distinct styles of yoga, the style familiar to most of us in the West is called *hatha yoga*. This style of yoga involves practicing a variety of static postures, or *asanas*. These postures stretch, strengthen, and align the body and increase flexibility. The practice of yoga also helps relieve physical and emotional stress and helps bring about a sense of inner peace, balance, and "oneness." To learn more about practicing yoga you can go to special classes in your neighborhood or learn positions from a video or book (*Yoga for Dummies* is a good book for beginners).

The MediterrAsian Balanced Meal System (MBMS)

For thousands of years the peoples of the Mediterranean region and Asia have never counted carbohydrate or fat grams, referred to a glycemic index, divided their food into blocks, or separated their food into proteins and starches. And they certainly haven't counted calories. Instead, they've simply eaten a wide variety of delicious foods until they felt full and satisfied. Yet the great majority of them managed to stay lean and fit. What can explain this extraordinary paradox?

Well, one reason could be that Mediterranean and Asian people have traditionally burned off some of the calories they consume by being physically active as part of their day-to-day lives. But there's another very important reason—*how they balance their meals*.

Instead of eating lots of high-calorie processed foods, red meats, and junk foods like we do in the West, the majority of foods Mediterranean and Asian people have traditionally eaten consists of minimally processed foods as close to their natural state as possible. These foods—vegetables, grains, legumes, fruits, and lean protein sources such as fish, poultry, and seafood—are all bulky, high in volume, and filling, but they are generally only low to moderate in calories. In simple terms, this means that if you eat a traditional Mediterranean- or Asian-style meal instead of a typical Western-style meal, you'll be able to eat *more* food while consuming *fewer* calories.

As an example, let's compare a Western-style meal, a Mediterranean-style meal, and an Asian-style meal (see the chart on page 95). How's that for a comparison? If you eat a traditionally balanced Mediterranean- or Asian-style meal instead of a typical burger and fries meal, you'll end up eating close to twice the volume of food but around half the calories. And unlike the burger and fries meal, the Mediterranean- and Asian-style meals aren't riddled with saturated and hydrogenated fat, sugar, and other nasties. Instead, they're overflowing with essential vitamins and minerals as well as many other health-giving nutrients and compounds such as phytochemicals, antioxidants, omega-3 fatty acids, and soluble and insoluble fibers.

WESTERN-STYLE MEAL	MEDITERRANEAN-STYLE MEAL	ASIAN-STYLE MEAL
1 quarter-pound burger with cheese	Sicilian salmon and pasta with roasted red pepper, zucchini, basil, and pine nuts	Bowl of fragrant broccoli and mushroom soup
1 large fries	1 slice crusty whole grain bread drizzled with [1/2] tablespoon extra virgin olive oil	Rice paper roll stuffed with chicken breast, snow pea sprouts, and peppers and served with a soy-sesame dipping sauce
	Large salad with tomatoes, olives, romaine lettuce, and red onion, served with olive oil and balsamic vinaigrette	Cantonese shrimp, cashew nut, and mixed vegetable stir-fry served over steamed long-grain rice
1 large soda	1 glass red wine	1 glass cold beer
1 ice cream sundae	Bowl of mixed berries served with a scoop of sorbet.	Fresh fruit salad with mango, lychees, and pineapple
Calories: 1,679	Calories: 860	Calories: 810

The Mediterranean- and Asian-style meals also boost your fat-fighting metabolism and ensure that your blood sugar levels stay balanced for sustained energy and concentration. And just as important, this food isn't only nutritious, it's also *delicious*, so your mind and senses will be satisfied too, which is incredibly important!

BALANCING ALL YOUR MEALS THIS WAY

How do you balance all your meals like the Mediterranean and Asian examples above so they're nutritious, filling, and delicious but only moderate in calories? Well, it's actually a lot easier than you may think. As a matter of fact, it's as easy as following these five simple steps when you prepare or purchase a meal:

Step 1 • Go with the grains.

Include a grain-based food such as rice, pasta, bread, noodles, bulgur, or couscous in each meal.

Step 2 • Value your vegetables.

Include a variety of colorful vegetables in each meal or have a salad or vegetable-based soup on the side.

Step 3 • Pick your protein.

Include a moderate amount of protein-based foods in each meal—preferably fish (any variety, but particularly fattier types of fish like salmon, tuna, mackerel, sardines, and anchovies, which are rich in omega-3) and seafood (such as shrimp, scallops, crab, oysters, clams, mussels, and squid), legumes (beans, peas, and lentils), nuts, or chicken. Use eggs sparingly and red meat (beef, pork, and lamb) only occasionally.

Step 4 • Favor the good fats.

Vegetable oils (particularly monounsaturated vegetable oils like olive, canola, and peanut oil) and fish oils (from the fish you eat) should make up the majority of fat in each meal. Dairy products such as cheese and yogurt can be used in moderate amounts, and butter should be used only occasionally or in very small amounts.

Step 5 • Savor the seasonings.

Use a variety of herbs, spices, condiments, and seasonings to add flavor, color, and depth to each meal.

We call this simple five-step meal preparation system the *MediterrAsian Balanced Meal System*, or MBMS for short. By using this simple yet powerful system, you'll never have to worry about not getting the right balance of food, because the MBMS is based directly on how Mediterranean and Asian people have instinctively been balancing their meals for thousands of years. So by designing your meals according to this system, you'll not only become leaner while eating lots of food, but you'll also automatically be following the healthiest diet in the world!

You can use the guidelines of the MBMS when you prepare your own meals or when you eat out, and it can even be used to adapt typically less healthy foods like burgers and hot dogs into far healthier versions that taste just as good. (We'll show you how shortly.)

USING THE MBMS IN REAL LIFE

It's easy to create a huge range of delicious and nutritious Mediterranean- and Asian-style meals using the guidelines of the MBMS. For example, by mixing and matching grains, vegetables, proteins, fats, and seasonings for the Mediterranean and Asian dishes listed below, it's possible to come up with literally thousands of different meal combinations.

PASTA DISHES

Go with the grains. Choose a type of pasta. It comes in more than four hundred varieties, but some of the most useful include spaghetti, lasagna, fusilli (corkscrew shape), fettuccine (flat, ribbonlike), penne (tubular with ends cut on diagonal), farfalle (bow-tie shape), and conchiglie (shells).

Value your vegetables. Tomatoes, onions, garlic, bell peppers (red, green, yellow, and orange), mushrooms, broccoli, zucchini, artichokes, arugula, celery, carrots, chiles, spinach, asparagus, and eggplant are some good choices.

Pick your protein. Good choices include tuna or salmon (fresh or canned), anchovies, fresh sardines, dried and fresh beans (cannellini beans, chickpeas, fresh green beans, and fava beans are particularly good choices), chicken, nuts (walnuts, pine nuts, and pistachios), and seafood like shrimp, crab, scallops, clams, mussels, squid, and octopus. Use meats like ground beef, salami, prosciutto, and pancetta only occasionally or in small amounts as a flavor and texture enhancer.

Favor the good fats. Use olive oil as your principal cooking fat. If you're having cheese with your pasta meal, opt for a strong-flavored variety like Parmesan so a little goes a long way.

Savor the seasonings. Sun-dried tomatoes, olives, vinegars (like balsamic and red wine), capers, red and white wine, basil, oregano, rosemary, flat-leaf parsley, sea salt, and freshly ground black pepper can all be used in various combinations.

For examples of MediterrAsian-balanced noodle dishes, see page 195.

STIR-FRIES

Go with the grains. A stir-fry is typically mixed or served with rice or noodles.

Value your vegetables. Broccoli, scallions, garlic, ginger, red and green bell peppers, zucchini, chili, celery, bean sprouts, cabbage (including Chinese cabbage), asparagus, cauliflower, carrots, mushrooms (fresh or dried), sweet corn, and Asian greens (such as bok choy, *gai lan*, and *choy sum*) are some good choices.

Pick your protein. Good choices include firm whitefish (like snapper, cod, and haddock), fresh tuna or salmon, tofu, chicken, nuts (almonds, cashews, or peanuts) and seafood like shrimp, crab (or surimi), squid, and scallops.

Favor the good fats. Use peanut or canola oil as your main cooking fat.

Savor the seasonings. Soy sauce, cilantro, five-spice powder, oyster sauce, rice wine, black bean sauce, hoisin sauce, and toasted sesame oil can all be used in various combinations.

For examples of MediterrAsian-balanced stir-fries, see page 155.

INDIAN CURRIES

Go with the grains. An Indian curry is typically served over rice (basmati is a good traditional variety) or with Indian breads such as *naan* or *chapati*.

Value your vegetables. Broccoli, cauliflower, garlic, ginger, tomatoes, carrots, scallions, eggplant, cucumber, cabbage, spinach, red and green bell peppers, and chilies are some good choices.

Pick your protein. Good choices include firm whitefish, salmon, tuna, chicken, lentils, chickpeas, almonds, green beans, fresh or dried peas, and seafood like shrimp and scallops.

Favor the good fats. Use peanut or canola oil as your cooking fat. Use only moderate amounts of coconut milk and yogurt.

Savor the seasonings. Fresh coriander and mint, tamarind, dried spices (including cumin, turmeric, coriander, cinnamon, and chili powder), and fruit and vegetable relishes and chutneys can all be used in various combinations.

For examples of MediterrAsian-balanced Indian curries, see page 171.

SUSHI ROLLS

Go with the grains. Rice is an integral part of sushi because it makes up the largest part of the filling. A short-grain rice is the best variety to use.

Value your vegetables. Nori (thin sheets of seaweed used to wrap sushi rolls), cucumber, bean sprouts, carrots, mushrooms (like shiitake and enoki), avocado, snow peas, and snow pea sprouts are some good choices.

Pick your protein. Good choices include very fresh raw salmon or tuna, smoked salmon, fish roe, tofu, and seafood like shrimp, squid, and crab (or use surimi as a crab substitute).

Favor the good fats. No fat or oil is used in the preparation of sushi, so the good fats come mainly from the omega-3 rich fish.

Savor the seasonings. Wasabi (hot Japanese horseradish paste), soy sauce, pickled ginger (*gari*), pickled radish (*daikon*), and rice vinegar are all possibilities.

For examples of MediterrAsian-balanced sushi rolls, see page 205.

Go with the grains. Choose a base for your pizza. Opt for either a premade pizza base (thin is traditional) or use large whole-grain pita bread as the base.

Value your vegetables. Tomato-based sauce and tomatoes, onion, garlic, bell peppers (red and green), mushrooms, eggplant, broccoli, zucchini, artichoke hearts, spinach, and asparagus are some good choices.

Pick your protein. Opt mainly for anchovies, tuna, smoked salmon, shrimp, scallops, smoked oysters, diced chicken, clams, and squid. We've also found that sliced soy hot dogs add a smoky sausage flavor to pizza without adding saturated fat. Use meaty toppings like ground beef, pepperoni, and salami only occasionally, or use them more as a garnish.

Favor the good fats. You can add flavor and texture to your pizza by drizzling the top with a little extra-virgin olive oil. Don't drown your pizza in cheese either, just lightly cover it—and use a good pizza cheese like mozzarella so you get both flavor and texture.

Savor the seasonings. Sun-dried tomatoes, olives (many varieties), capers, basil, oregano, rosemary, flat-leaf parsley, sea salt, and freshly ground black pepper can all be used in various combinations.

MEDITERRASIAN MAKEOVERS

The examples above show you how the MBMS can be used to create lots of different traditional Mediterranean and Asian dishes. But it's not only Mediterranean and Asian meals that can be put together using the guidelines of the MBMS. Many Western-style meals can also be easily adapted to follow MBMS guidelines. Following are some examples.

BURGERS

Burgers have gotten a very bad reputation for being unhealthy and fattening. But when you think about it, if you remove the meat patty from a burger with cheese, what you're left with is basically a cheese and salad roll. So the key to making a burger far healthier is to find a healthy yet tasty alternative to the meat patty. You can also add more bulk, flavor, and nutrients to the burger by including more vegetables (which are naturally *very* low in calories).

Go with the grains. Choose a burger bun, regular or whole grain.

Value your vegetables. Fill your burger with lots of vegetables, including thinly sliced onions, tomatoes, lettuce, and pickles.

Pick your protein. Instead of using a beef patty to make your burger, opt for a soy, lentil, bean, fish, or chicken-based patty.

Favor the good fats. Cook the burger patties in a little canola, peanut, or light olive oil. If you add mayonnaise to your burger, use it more sparingly and preferably use an olive oil– or canola oil–based mayo. If you're having cheese with your burger, use a sharp cheese such as cheddar so a little goes a long way.

Savor the seasonings. Add flavor to your burger with condiments and sauces like ketchup, mustard (many varieties), BBQ sauce, relish, chutney, salsa, chili sauce, pepper, or horseradish.

SANDWICHES AND SUBS

By making a few sensible choices when you're constructing a sandwich, you can easily keep the calories down while increasing the bulk and the flavor—in other words, you can eat a bigger, tastier sandwich while consuming fewer calories!

Go with the grains. Choose a bread, preferably a whole-grain variety. Vary the type of bread you use—some examples include sliced whole-grain bread, pita bread, Middle Eastern lavash bread, rolls (many different types), French baguettes, Italian breads (like focaccia or ciabatta), or Turkish *pide* bread.

Value your vegetables. Pack your sandwich with a generous serving of any combination of salad vegetables you like—lettuce (iceberg, romaine, or other varieties), tomatoes, onions, bell peppers (red, green, orange, or yellow), carrots, sprouts (such as alfalfa, bean, or snow pea), cucumber, celery, sweet corn kernels, mushrooms, scallions, and char-grilled and marinated vegetables such as eggplant, peppers, or zucchini.

Pick your protein. Use red meat and meat products on your sandwich only occasionally. Opt instead for canned tuna, salmon (canned or smoked), mashed canned sardines, roast chicken or turkey, shrimp (fresh or canned), crab (or surimi), or soy-based ham and bacon. Canned beans are another versatile and healthy high-protein sandwich filling. Hard-boiled eggs can be used in moderation.

Favor the good fats. Spread your bread lightly with canola oil– or olive oil–based margarine (preferably trans-fat free). You can also use avocado or hummus. If you add mayonnaise to your sub or sandwich, use it more sparingly (the same goes for other creamy dressings such as seafood cocktail sauce). And if you have cheese on your sandwich, use a strong variety like sharp cheddar so a little goes a long way.

Savor the seasonings. To add extra flavor to your sandwich, there are plenty of condiments to choose from—mustard (lots of varieties), olives, chutney, relish, horseradish, salsa, pickles, sun-dried tomatoes, cranberry sauce, pesto, sweet chili sauce, freshly ground black pepper, lemon juice, and vinegar are some good examples.

HOT DOGS

A normal hot dog is simply oozing with saturated fat. But you can enjoy all the wonderful flavors of a hot dog without any of the guilt by applying the guidelines of the MBMS.

Go with the grains. Choose a hot dog roll, regular or whole grain.

Value your vegetables. As well as onions, there are lots of other vegetables you can add to hot dogs, including sautéed red and green bell peppers, mushrooms, and garlic. Alternatively, have a serving of coleslaw with your hot dog.

Pick your protein. Instead of using a meat-based hot dog, opt for a soy-based hot dog.

Favor the good fats. The best way to cook a hot dog is in the microwave or in plenty of hot boiling water, so fat isn't required in the cooking process. By eating a soy-based hot dog instead of a meat-based one, you're already favoring the good fats. If you have cheese on your hot dog, use a strong variety like sharp cheddar so a little goes a long way.

Savor the seasonings. Add flavor to your hot dog with condiments and sauces like ketchup, mustard (many varieties), BBQ sauce, chili sauce, relish, salsa, and chutney.

BARBECUES

At a typical Western barbecue the focus is squarely on the meat. A MediterrAsian-balanced barbecue, on the other hand, divides the focus between the grilled food and the bread and side dishes.

Go with the grains. Serve bread (such as sliced whole-grain bread, pita, lavash, ciabatta, or baguette) or bread rolls on the side.

Value your vegetables. Have a salad on the side, add vegetable pieces to kebabs, or cook up some vegetables on the grill (bell peppers, onion, eggplant, mushrooms, and zucchini grill particularly well).

Pick your protein. Instead of the usual steak and sausages, opt mainly for salmon, tuna or swordfish steaks, or soy-based sausages. Other alternatives include soy-, fish-, or chicken-based burger patties; any kind of firm fresh fish; and seafood like shrimp, squid, scallops, and mussels.

Favor the good fats. Use canola oil, peanut oil, or olive oil as your cooking fat. Instead of serving bread with butter or margarine, have a small dish of extra-virgin olive oil for dipping or drizzling. Alternatively, use a trans fat–free margarine made from olive or canola oil.

Savor the seasonings. Add flavor to the grilled food either with a marinade (which can be used for basting and marinating) or with condiments and sauces like ketchup, mustard (many varieties), barbecue sauce, relish, salsa, and chutney.

EATING OUT: A WORLD OF CHOICE

One of the joys of eating MediterrAsian-balanced meals is that you don't have to prepare them all at home. We enjoy going out to restaurants and getting takeout meals weekly while still applying the principles of the MBMS—here's how we do it.

Restaurants

Without a doubt, dining out should be a highly pleasurable experience. Why spend good money at a restaurant and leave feeling unsatisfied? Why spend an evening out with friends if you can't enjoy the pleasure of eating with everyone else?

Eating a MediterrAsian-balanced meal when you dine out at a restaurant is incredibly simple. Actually, we're willing to bet that a lot of your favorite restaurant food is already based on Mediterranean and Asian cuisine. Think of the countries of the Mediterranean region and Asia, and you can probably match it up with a favorite restaurant. Some examples include Italian, Indian, Greek, Thai, Chinese, Lebanese, French Provençal, Vietnamese, Turkish, and Japanese. And these restaurants often have a takeout section, and many even deliver, so you can also enjoy these foods in the comfort of your own home.

But just because a meal is from a Mediterranean- or Asian-style restaurant doesn't necessarily mean it will be MediterrAsian-balanced. Many of the meals in these restaurants are actually based on the banquet foods that are eaten in these countries and not necessarily on the staple meals that are eaten by people every day. That's why many people who dine out regularly at these restaurants wonder why they gain weight—Mediterranean and Asian people would most certainly gain weight too if they ate banquet foods every day!

At the same time, many Mediterranean and Asian restaurants have adapted their meals for a Western palate. In other words, now there's usually lots of red meat, fried food, and cream-style sauces on the menu.

With all that said, you should still have no problem finding lots of dishes in Mediterranean and Asian-style restaurants that will be traditionally balanced—it's just a matter of looking. If you keep in mind the guidelines of the MBMS when you're reviewing the menu, it will make things a lot easier.

Here are some good examples of what types of meals to keep an eye out for at various Mediterranean- and Asian-style restaurants:

ITALIAN

Pasta dishes with fish, shellfish, chicken, or legumes and vegetables served with a tomato-based sauce like marinara or pomodoro or an olive oil– and herb-based sauce like pesto or *salsa verde*

Thin-base pizza (which is traditional) topped with vegetables and different kinds of fish and shellfish, like anchovies, salmon, shrimp or clams

Vegetable-, seafood-, chicken-, or bean-based risotto

Grilled fish, poultry, or vegetables served with rice, pasta, polenta (cornmeal), or bread and salad

Fish, shellfish, chicken, vegetable, or bean dishes cooked in tomato-, wine-, or
stock-based sauces served with ciabatta or focaccia bread on the side
Vegetable- or legume-based salads served with olive oil vinaigrette
Vegetable-, fish-, shellfish-, poultry-, or bean-based soups
Bruschetta (garlic and olive oil toasts) topped with grilled or roasted vegetables
(like tomatoes and peppers) and drizzled with a little olive oil
Antipasti (appetizers), such as marinated vegetables, olives, sun-dried tomatoes,
and small amounts of cheese and cold meat (like shaved ham or salami)
A fruit platter, or gelato served with fresh fruit

GREEK AND MIDDLE EASTERN

Fish, shellfish, poultry, vegetables, or legumes cooked in sauces based on wine,
stock, tomato, and yogurt
Traditional Greek salad (*horiatiki*) with tomatoes, cucumbers, feta cheese,
kalamata olives, and red onion
Fish, shellfish, or poultry grilled, baked, or poached with onions, tomatoes,
peppers, garlic, and other vegetables and served over rice or bulgur
Grape leaves stuffed with rice, vegetables, and pine nuts or pistachios
Legume, fish, shellfish, or poultry-based pilaf
Meze (traditional Greek and Middle Eastern appetizer dishes similar to Italian
antipasto)
Chicken-, falafel-, or seafood-based gyros served with salad
Pita bread stuffed with grilled chicken, falafel, or shrimp and vegetables
Tabbouleh (tomato, bulgur, parsley, and mint salad)
Fish-, shellfish-, poultry-, or legume-based pasta dishes
Vegetable-, bean-, or lentil-based soups
Crusty bread sticks or pita bread dipped into baba ghanoush (smoky eggplant
dip), hummus (chickpea and sesame dip), or *tzatziki* (yogurt-cucumber dip)
Rice pudding served with fruit and crushed nuts

FRENCH PROVENÇAL

Niçoise salad (with tuna, tomatoes, potatoes, olives, sliced boiled eggs,
and lettuce)
Bouillabaisse (fish and shellfish stew)
Pan bagnat (bread stuffed with Niçoise salad)
Crêpes stuffed with fish, shellfish, poultry, or beans
Toasted baguette spread with *tapenade* (olive, garlic, and caper spread)
Roasted, grilled, or stuffed eggplant, and artichokes, zucchini, and tomatoes

Vegetable, bean, or lentil soups (such as *soupe au pistou*)

Ratatouille (a vegetable stew traditionally made with tomatoes, bell pepper, eggplant, and zucchini; it goes wonderfully served on the side of grilled or baked fish, chicken, or shellfish)

Salade verte (green salad served with any combination of fresh leaves, including endive, arugula, spinach, or watercress) dressed with vinaigrette

Grilled, broiled, steamed, roasted fish, shellfish, or chicken dishes

Crudités (fresh raw vegetable pieces) with white bean dip

Fresh fruits in liqueur like Cointreau or Grand Marnier

Fruit-filled crêpes

SPANISH

Paella (saffron-infused rice dish with any combination of seafood, chicken, beans, and vegetables)

Tortilla de patatas (an egg dish with potatoes, similar to an omelet)

Tapas, small appetizer dishes (which could include garlic shrimp, steamed mussels, fried squid, marinated mushrooms and artichokes, olives, or roasted marinated red peppers)

Vegetable soups like gazpacho (chilled tomato and cucumber soup) and seafood soups (which include mussels, shrimp, or fish)

Tomato-based stews made with fish, shellfish, or beans and vegetables like potatoes, bell peppers, or zucchini

Grilled tuna or salmon skewers with vegetables (such as mixed peppers, tomatoes, red onions, potatoes) and Spanish-style tomato sauce

Chickpea salad with roasted peppers and capers

Hogazas (thick slices of bread with toppings like tomato, ham, red peppers, or anchovies)

Bean stews made with any combination of white beans, fava beans, or chickpeas

Vegetable, bean, or seafood soup served with crusty bread

Fruit compotes using fruit such as plums, cherries, apricots, or peaches

NORTH AFRICAN (INCLUDING MOROCCAN AND TUNISIAN)

Tagine (stew) made with combinations of fish, beans (like chickpeas), chicken, vegetables, nuts, fruits, herbs, and spices served over couscous

Soups made with vegetables, chickpeas, and lentils

North African baked fish flavored with *chermoula* (Moroccan spice mixture) and served with vegetables and rice or couscous

Salads like couscous and vegetable salad, orange and black olive salad, carrot salad, or bean salad

Bean dips like *ful nabed* (lima bean puree) and *bessara* (white bean dip) served with pita bread

Vegetables (like peppers and eggplants) stuffed with couscous (or rice) nuts and vegetables

Chakchouka (a North African cousin of Provençal ratatouille—a mixture of peppers, onions, and tomatoes fried in olive oil with herbs, spices, and eggs)

Seafood or chicken *bastilla*—a spiced phyllo pastry pie

Sweet couscous with almonds, honey, cinnamon, and dried or fresh fruits

Oranges with dates, pistachio nuts, rosewater, and cinnamon

SOUTHEAST ASIAN (INCLUDING THAI, VIETNAMESE, MALAYSIAN, AND INDONESIAN CUISINE)

Steamed, grilled, poached, or baked fish, shellfish, poultry, tempeh, or tofu dishes served over rice or noodles

Vegetable, fish, or shellfish soups like *Tom yum goong* (Thai hot and sour shrimp soup) or *Soto Ayam* (spicy Malaysian chicken soup)

Red, green, or yellow Thai curry with vegetables and fish, shellfish, poultry, or tofu served over steamed or boiled rice

Steamed spring rolls filled with shrimp, chicken, or crab and vegetables

Vietnamese-style fresh rice paper rolls filled with vegetables and chicken or seafood

Indonesian satay (marinated skewers) with chicken, fish, or shellfish

Gado gado (cooked vegetable salad with peanut sauce)

Kha Phat (Thai fried rice) with shrimp, crab, tofu, chicken, or squid

Pad Thai (stir-fried noodle, shrimp, and vegetable dish)

Nasi goreng (Indonesian fried rice) with chicken or seafood and vegetables

Mie goreng (Indonesian fried noodles) with chicken or seafood and vegetables

Laksa (Malaysian spicy noodle soup) with fish, shellfish, tofu, or chicken and vegetables

INDIAN

Fish-, shellfish-, chicken-, lentil-, or chickpea-based curries served over rice and accompanied with relish, chutney, and raita (yogurt and cucumber)

Dahl (lentil curry) served over rice or accompanied with breads like naan or chapati

Fish, chicken, or shrimp cooked Tandoori style (marinated and baked) or *vindoori* style (marinated and braised) and served over rice or with bread

Lentil-, bean-, fish-, shellfish-, and vegetable-based soups

Vegetable-based curries like pea and potato curry served over rice with naan or chapati bread

Vegetable-based salads like *tamatar salat* (tomato salad with mint and scallions)

Pilau (a rice dish similar to a Middle Eastern pilaf) made with vegetables and fish, shellfish, or beans like chickpeas

Grilled, baked, or poached fish, shellfish, or chicken served in tomato-, yogurt-, or stock-based sauces

Murgh Tikka (skewered barbecued chicken) served with rice and a vegetable side dish

CHINESE

Stir-fried seafood, fish, chicken, or tofu (called bean curd in China) and vegetables served over rice or noodles

Soups such as crab and sweet corn soup, chicken noodle soup, or hot and sour soup

Chow mein made with vegetables and either fish, shellfish, tofu, or chicken (or a combination)

Roasted lemon chicken served with vegetables over rice

Fried rice made with shrimp (or other shellfish), fish, or chicken and vegetables

Braised fish, shellfish, tofu, or chicken with vegetables served over rice or noodles

Fish, vegetables, shellfish, or tofu with sweet and sour sauce served over rice or noodles

Steamed spring rolls and wontons filled with vegetables and seafood or chicken

Steamed shrimp or chicken dumplings

Noodle salad in sesame sauce

Fresh fruit and fortune cookies

JAPANESE

Yaki (broiled or grilled) or *nimono* (simmered) dishes with fish, shellfish, or chicken and vegetables served with rice or noodles (udon or soba)

Sashimi (thinly sliced raw fish such as tuna, salmon, whitefish, or mackerel) served with rice and vegetables on the side

Sushi made with vegetables and your choice of fish and shellfish

Light soups like miso or *sakana ushiojiru* (fish broth)

Heavier noodle-based soups like *yosenabe* (simmered seafood, vegetable, and noodle soup)

Steamed rice and noodles topped with vegetables and fish, tofu, or chicken

Teriyaki salmon, tuna, shellfish, or chicken served with vegetables and rice or noodles

Tempura (lightly breaded and deep-fried seafood and vegetables) is good in moderation

Hot or cold soba (buckwheat) noodles with vegetables and seafood

Fresh fruit platter

Fast-Food Outlets

Restaurant cuisine isn't the only type of food you can enjoy when you eat out. Armed with your knowledge of the MBMS, it's also possible to eat at popular Western fast-food outlets.

PIZZA

The great thing about ordering a pizza is that you can add or take away ingredients. This means it's quite possible to turn a Western-style pizza into more of a MediterrAsian-balanced meal. The key is to load up on the vegetables and choose healthy protein sources with your pizza. So instead of going for the meat-lovers pizza, opt instead for the seafood-lovers pizza. Beans and chicken are also good high-protein toppings.

Also opt for the traditional Italian thin-based pizza instead of the Western pan-pizza, which contains far more calories in the crust.

Fast-food pizza outlets also tend to go overboard with the cheese, so when you order your pizza tell them to halve the cheese and double the vegetables. This will make the pizza more flavorful and filling while keeping the calories and saturated fat down. A fresh salad with an olive oil-based dressing is also a good accompaniment to pizza.

BURGERS

When you eat a burger at a fast food outlet, no matter how much you try to balance it, it's still going to be a high-calorie treat. But there are ways of minimizing the damage and making the burger more MediterrAsian-balanced.

For a start you could opt for a chicken- or fish-based burger instead of a beef-based one; this will reduce your intake of saturated fat and calories. A Filet-O-Fish, for example, contains less than half the saturated fat of a Big Mac, and a Premium Grilled

Chicken Classic Sandwich contains less than a quarter of the saturated fat. Fish- and chicken-based burgers also generally contain between 150 and 250 calories fewer than a typical beef-based burger. And make sure to order a burger that comes with lots of salad veggies, including lettuce, tomatoes, onions, and pickles. These not only make the burger more filling and tasty but add essential vitamins and minerals.

French fries also contain lots of calories as well as bad fat, so consume these foods in moderation. (In other words, order the small fries instead of the large fries.)

SANDWICHES AND SUBS

Sandwich shops and delis are some of the easiest places to get a quick MediterrAsian-balanced meal because the sandwich is constructed according to your own wishes. This means that all you have to do is follow the guidelines for making your own MediterrAsian-balanced subs and sandwiches at home (see page 101). The only difference is that someone else is conveniently making it for you in the deli, and you don't have to shop for the ingredients.

So far we've talked about how to balance your meals according to the MBMS. But it's very important to remember that all your meals don't have to be MediterrAsian-balanced. As long as it's in moderation, sometimes an unbalanced meal like a beef burger or fried chicken is fine. However, if you try to make the majority of your meals MediterrAsian-balanced—or at least try to follow as many of the five steps as possible—the health-giving benefits will be far more substantial.

And you'll find that because MediterrAsian-style food is so delicious and filling, it really doesn't make sense to cheat much, because it feels like you're cheating the whole time anyway!

A 14-Day Example
of MediterrAsian Living

In our opinion, most diets are destined to fail in the long run for two main reasons: *deprivation* and *complication*. No matter how much a diet will try to cover up the fact that it's depriving you, deep down they all are—whether it's depriving you of fat, or carbohydrates, or simply food.

What's your first reaction when you're deprived of something? You end up wanting it twice as much, don't you? At the same time, it takes steely discipline to stay on a diet because, invariably, they're complicated and time-consuming.

But compare this to how the peoples of the Mediterranean region and Asia having been living for the past few thousand years. Instead of strict diets, they've simply eaten lots of good food until they felt full and satisfied; instead of grueling exercise routines they've simply moved as a consequence of their everyday lives; and they've also made sure to set aside time each day to relax and rejuvenate—by themselves and with the company of friends and loved ones. Talk about the total opposite of deprivation and complication! And we truly believe it's this *healthy balanced lifestyle*—incorporating wholesome food, natural movement, and emotional calm time—that equates to a healthy body, mind, and spirit and lays down solid foundations for achieving a long, disease-free life.

THE FOURTEEN-DAY PLAN

To give you an example of how to incorporate this healthy balanced lifestyle into your own life, we've designed a fourteen-day plan based on how we live day to day. The plan includes all the meals, snacks, and drinks for a full fourteen days, and it also includes lots of tips and ideas on how you can easily incorporate natural movement and calm time into your daily life.

It's important to remember that this is just an example of how to live. If you want to follow it to the letter, that's up to you—but we think a far better approach is to mix and match the meals and adapt the plan to fit into your own life and your own circumstances. And speaking of fitting a MediterrAsian lifestyle into different circumstances, in the next chapter we'll show you just how easily you can adapt this way of living to any situation—from busy workdays and hectic weekends, to when you're at a party, on vacation, or traveling at thirty thousand feet.

Day 1

Breakfast
- A bowl of whole-grain breakfast cereal (for example, oatmeal, Bran Flakes®, Wheaties®, All-Bran®, Shredded Wheat®, untoasted muesli, or wheat-biscuit cereals such as Weet-bix® and Weetabix®) with soy or regular milk

Lunch
- Sandwich or 6-inch sub sandwich on whole-grain bread (homemade or store-bought): tuna, chicken, crab, or turkey with lettuce, tomatoes, sliced onions, cucumber, grated carrot, peppers, or other vegetables and mustard, mayo, olives, pickles, and preserved chili as flavor enhancers
- 1 fresh peach

Dinner
- Pesto Chicken Pizza (page 170)

Dessert
- 2 sliced kiwi fruit topped with a scoop of your favorite ice cream

Snacks
- Choose 3 separate snacks from the MediterrAsian-Friendly Snacks list on page 126 and enjoy them throughout the day between meals.

Beverages
- 1 to 2 cups of tea or coffee
- 1 to 2 glasses of wine or beer
- Plenty of water

Natural Movement
- Be physically active for at least 30 minutes. Choose from the Natural Movement ideas on page 68, or come up with your own.

Calm Time
- Physically and emotionally relax for at least 20 minutes. Choose from the Calm Time ideas on page 87, or come up with your own.

Day 2

Breakfast
- Half a medium can of baked beans, heated and served on two slices of lightly buttered whole-grain toast
- 1 fresh orange

Lunch
- Savory Salmon Spread Sandwich: Spread 2 tablespoons of Savory Salmon Spread (page 290) on a slice of whole-grain bread. Top with 4 sliced cucumber rounds and half a cup of shredded lettuce. Sandwich together with another slice of whole-grain bread and cut in half to serve.
- A small bunch of grapes

Dinner
- Lemony Tuna, Olive, and Vegetable Pasta (page 146)

Dessert
- Pears with Peach Ricotta Whip and Almonds (page 294)

Snacks
- Choose 3 separate snacks from the MediterrAsian-Friendly Snacks list on page 126, and enjoy them throughout the day between meals.

Beverages
- 1 to 2 cups of tea or coffee
- 1 to 2 glasses of wine or beer
- Plenty of water

Natural Movement
- Be physically active for at least 20 minutes. Choose from the Natural Movement ideas on page 68, or come up with your own.

Calm Time
- Physically and emotionally relax for at least 30 minutes. Choose from the Calm Time ideas on page 87, or come up with your own.

Day 3

Breakfast
- Tomato and cheese toasts: Toast two slices of whole-grain bread and melt a little sliced cheese on top, then arrange some sliced tomato on top and garnish with salt and freshly ground black pepper.
- 1 apple

Lunch
- Hummus and Salad Wraps (page 233)
- 6 dried apricots

Dinner
- Mushroom, Bacon, and Walnut Risotto (page 189)

Dessert
- A cup of strawberries topped with ½ cup of your favorite fruit yogurt

Snacks
- Choose 3 snacks from the MediterrAsian-Friendly Snacks list on page 126, and enjoy them throughout the day between meals.

Beverages
- 1 to 2 cups of tea or coffee
- 1 to 2 glasses of wine or beer
- A glass of freshly squeezed juice
- Plenty of water

Natural Movement
- Be physically active for at least 20 minutes. Choose from the Natural Movement ideas on page 68, or come up with your own.

Calm Time
- Physically and emotionally relax for at least 30 minutes. Choose from the Calm Time ideas on page 87, or come up with your own.

Day 4

Breakfast	• Creamy Fruit and Nut Oatmeal (page 266)
Lunch	• Chicken salad sandwich: Combine 5 ounces (150 g) shredded cooked chicken breast with sliced tomato, shredded lettuce, sliced cucumber, and a tablespoon of mayo on multigrain bread (2 slices). • ¼ small cantaloupe
Dinner	• Shrimp, Bok Choy, and Snow Pea Stir-Fry (page 159)
Dessert	• 1 sliced banana topped with a scoop of your favorite ice cream
Snacks	• Choose 3 separate snacks from the MediterrAsian-Friendly Snacks list on page 126, and enjoy them throughout the day between meals.
Beverages	• 1 to 2 cups of tea or coffee • 1 to 2 glasses of wine or beer • Plenty of water
Natural Movement	• Be physically active for at least 20 minutes. Choose from the Natural Movement ideas on page 68, or come up with your own.
Calm Time	• Physically and emotionally relax for at least 30 minutes. Choose from the Calm Time ideas on page 87, or come up with your own.

Day 5

Breakfast	• Sardine Toast Topper (page 265) • 1 tangerine
Lunch	• Go to a sushi bar and order 10 pieces of sushi and a bowl of miso soup; finish with a simple fresh fruit salad.
Dinner	• Moroccan Stew with Couscous (page 181)
Dessert	• Tunisian Date, Orange, and Pistachio Salad (page 295)
Snacks	• Choose 3 separate snacks from the MediterrAsian-Friendly Snacks list on page 126, and enjoy them throughout the day between meals.
Beverages	• 1 to 2 cups of tea or coffee • 1 to 2 glasses of wine or beer • Plenty of water
Natural Movement	• Be physically active for at least 20 minutes. Choose from the Natural Movement ideas on page 68, or come up with your own.
Calm Time	• Physically and emotionally relax for at least 30 minutes. Choose from the Calm Time ideas on page 87, or come up with your own.

Day 6

Breakfast
- Italian-Style Scrambled Eggs (page 264)
- A small handful of cherries

Lunch
- Savory Tuna Melt: Toast 2 slices of whole-grain bread, then top each slice with 2 tablespoons of Savory Tuna Spread (page 290) and a little sliced cheddar cheese. Place under a hot broiler for a minute, or until the cheese is bubbling and golden brown.
- 6 dried apricots

Dinner
- Night out at a Mediterranean- or Asian-style restaurant (Greek, Italian, Chinese, Spanish, Japanese, Indian, Thai, or Moroccan):
  Order traditional dishes based around fish, seafood, chicken, legumes, grains, and vegetables.

Dessert
- Choose a fruit-based dessert.

Snacks
- Choose 3 separate snacks from the MediterrAsian-Friendly Snacks list on page 126, and enjoy them throughout the day between meals.

Beverages
- 1 to 2 cups of tea or coffee
- 1 to 2 glasses of wine or beer
- Plenty of water

Natural Movement
- Be physically active for at least 20 minutes. Choose from the Natural Movement ideas on page 68, or come up with your own.

Calm Time
- Physically and emotionally relax for at least 30 minutes. Choose from the Calm Time ideas on page 87, or come up with your own.

Day 7

Breakfast
- Peanut butter on toast: Toast two slices of whole-grain bread and top each slice with 2 teaspoons of natural peanut butter.
- 1 nectarine

Lunch
- Chicken and Avocado Salad Wraps: Spread 1 tablespoon of mayonnaise in a horizontal line down the middle of a whole-grain flat bread (such as pocketless pita bread or a flour tortilla). Arrange ½ cup of shredded precooked chicken breast, ½ cup of torn iceberg lettuce, ¼ of a sliced avocado, 1 tablespoon of finely chopped green bell pepper and ½ of a sliced tomato evenly on top. Season with salt and pepper and roll up.
- 2 kiwi fruit

Dinner
- Salmon Kedgeree (page 190)

Dessert
- 1 sliced banana topped with ½ cup of your favorite fruit yogurt

Snacks
- Choose 3 separate snacks from the MediterrAsian-Friendly Snacks list on page 126, and enjoy them throughout the day between meals.

Beverages
- 1 to 2 cups of tea or coffee
- 1 to 2 glasses of wine or beer
- Plenty of water

Natural Movement
- Be physically active for at least 20 minutes. Choose from the Natural Movement ideas on page 68, or come up with your own.

Calm Time
- Physically and emotionally relax for at least 30 minutes. Choose from the Calm Time ideas on page 87, or come up with your own.

Day 8

Breakfast	• Bruschetta with Tomato, Mozzarella, and Anchovy (page 236) • 1 sliced apple
Lunch	• Savory Tuna Spread Sandwich: Spread 2 tablespoons of Savory Tuna Spread (page 290) on a slice of multigrain bread. Top with 4 sliced cucumber rounds and half a cup of shredded lettuce. Sandwich together with another slice of multigrain bread and cut in half to serve. • 3 plums
Dinner	• Stir-Fried Tofu, Vegetables, and Water Chestnuts in Oyster Sauce (page 157)
Dessert	• Asian-Style Fruit Salad (page 296)
Snacks	• Choose 3 separate snacks from the MediterrAsian-Friendly Snacks list on page 126, and enjoy them throughout the day between meals.
Beverages	• 1 to 2 cups of tea or coffee • 1 to 2 glasses of wine or beer • A glass of freshly squeezed juice • Plenty of water
Natural Movement	• Be physically active for at least 20 minutes. Choose from the Natural Movement ideas on page 68, or come up with your own.
Calm Time	• Physically and emotionally relax for at least 30 minutes. Choose from the Calm Time ideas on page 87, or come up with your own.

Day 9

Breakfast
- A bowl of whole-grain breakfast cereal (for example, oatmeal, Bran Flakes®, Wheaties®, All-Bran®, Shredded Wheat®, untoasted muesli, or wheat-biscuit cereals such as Weet-bix® and Weetabix®) with soy or regular milk
- 1 pear

Lunch
- Curried Egg and Salad Sandwich: In a small bowl mash 1 hard-boiled egg with a fork and stir in ½ tablespoon of mayonnaise, ¼ teaspoon of curry powder, and a pinch each of salt and pepper until well combined. Spread the curried egg mixture evenly over 1 slice of whole-grain bread and top with ½ cup shredded lettuce and half a grated carrot. Sandwich together with another whole-grain bread slice and cut in half to serve.
- 1 mandarin

Dinner
- Sicilian Tuna and Basil Pizza (page 163)

Dessert
- Strawberry and blueberry fruit salad: Combine 6 hulled sliced strawberries, ¼ cup of blueberries, 1 teaspoon of sugar, and a tablespoon of water in a bowl. Toss together and serve with a scoop of your favorite ice cream.

Snacks
- Choose 3 separate snacks from the MediterrAsian-Friendly Snacks list on page 126, and enjoy them throughout the day between meals.

Beverages
- 1 to 2 cups of tea or coffee
- 1 to 2 glasses of wine or beer
- Plenty of water

Natural Movement
- Be physically active for at least 20 minutes. Choose from the Natural Movement ideas on page 68, or come up with your own.

Calm Time
- Physically and emotionally relax for at least 30 minutes. Choose from the Calm Time ideas on page 87, or come up with your own.

Day 10

Breakfast
- Half a medium can of baked beans served on two slices of lightly buttered whole-grain toast
- 1 orange

Lunch
- Sandwich or 6-inch sub on whole-grain bread (homemade or store-bought): tuna, chicken, crab, or turkey with lettuce, tomatoes, sliced onions, cucumber, grated carrot, peppers, or other vegetables and mustard, mayo, olives, pickles, and preserved chili as flavor enhancers.
- 1 banana

Dinner
- Thai Red Chicken Curry (page 172)

Dessert
- Mango with Lime Syrup and Toasted Coconut (page 293)

Snacks
- Choose 3 separate snacks from the MediterrAsian-Friendly Snacks list on page 126, and enjoy them throughout the day between meals.

Beverages
- 1 to 2 cups of tea or coffee
- 1 to 2 glasses of wine or beer
- Plenty of water

Natural Movement
- Be physically active for at least 20 minutes. Choose from the Natural Movement ideas on page 68, or come up with your own.

Calm Time
- Physically and emotionally relax for at least 30 minutes. Choose from the Calm Time ideas on page 87, or come up with your own.

Day 11

Breakfast	• A bowl of oatmeal topped with ½ chopped apple and a sprinkle of cinnamon
	• 1 tangerine
Lunch	• Greek Salad Pita Pockets (page 234)
	• 2 fresh apricots
Dinner	• Pasta Puttanesca (page 144)
Dessert	• Fruit and Nut Platter: Combine ½ sliced apple, 2 dried figs, a handful of grapes, 6 walnut halves, and 10 almonds on a platter.
Snacks	• Choose 3 separate snacks from the MediterrAsian-Friendly Snacks list on page 126, and enjoy them throughout the day between meals.
Beverages	• 1 to 2 cups of tea or coffee
	• 1 to 2 glasses of wine or beer
	• Plenty of water
Natural Movement	• Be physically active for at least 20 minutes. Choose from the Natural Movement ideas on page 68, or come up with your own.
Calm Time	• Physically and emotionally relax for at least 30 minutes. Choose from the Calm Time ideas on page 87, or come up with your own.

Day 12

Breakfast	• A bowl of whole-grain breakfast cereal (for example, oatmeal, Bran Flakes®, Wheaties®, All-Bran®, Shredded Wheat®, untoasted muesli, or wheat-biscuit cereals such as Weet-bix® and Weetabix®) with soy or regular milk, topped with strawberries or blueberries
Lunch	• Italian-Style Hot Dogs (page 229) • 1 banana
Dinner	• Salad plate with canned salmon: Arrange 5 ounces (150 g) of canned Alaskan salmon on a plate with 1 tomato (cut into wedges), 10 cucumber slices, a handful of your favorite lettuce, ½ grated carrot, 6 kalamata olives, and 4 red onion slices. Drizzle the vegetables with a tablespoon each of balsamic vinegar and extra-virgin olive oil, and season with sea salt and freshly ground black pepper. Serve with a thick slice of crusty whole-grain bread on the side.
Dessert	• Strawberries and Mascarpone Cheese (page 296)
Snacks	• Choose 3 separate snacks from the MediterrAsian-Friendly Snacks list on page 126, and enjoy them throughout the day between meals.
Beverages	• 1 to 2 cups of tea or coffee • 1 to 2 glasses of wine or beer • Plenty of water
Natural Movement	• Be physically active for at least 20 minutes. Choose from the Natural Movement ideas on page 68, or come up with your own.
Calm Time	• Physically and emotionally relax for at least 30 minutes. Choose from the Calm Time ideas on page 87, or come up with your own.

Day 13

Breakfast
- Tuna, Pea, and Corn Frittata (page 262)
- 1 orange

Lunch
- Vegetable and almond soup: Heat up ½ can of good-quality, store-bought vegetable soup; when warm, transfer to a blender and add 2 tablespoons of almond meal, blend, then reheat and serve in a bowl with a thick slice of whole-grain country bread.
- 1 peach

Dinner
- Night out at a Mediterranean- or Asian-style restaurant (Greek, Italian, Chinese, Spanish, Japanese, Indian, Thai, and Moroccan). Order traditional dishes based around fish, seafood, chicken, legumes, grains, and vegetables.

Dessert
- Choose a fruit-based dessert.

Snacks
- Choose 3 separate snacks from the MediterrAsian-Friendly Snacks list on page 126, and enjoy them throughout the day between meals.

Beverages
- 1 to 2 cups of tea or coffee
- 1 to 2 glasses of wine or beer
- Plenty of water

Natural Movement
- Be physically active for at least 20 minutes. Choose from the Natural Movement ideas on page 68, or come up with your own.

Calm Time
- Physically and emotionally relax for at least 30 minutes. Choose from the Calm Time ideas on page 87, or come up with your own.

Day 14

Breakfast	• Smoked Salmon and Avocado Bagels (page 267) • A handful of cherries
Lunch	• Ham salad sandwich: Combine a thin slice of ham with sliced tomato, shredded lettuce, a little diced red onion, and a teaspoon of your favorite mustard on lightly buttered multigrain bread (2 slices). • 1 nectarine
Dinner	• Japanese-Style Grilled Marinated Tuna (page 216) with Japanese Soba Noodle Salad (page 252)
Dessert	• Mango, Grape, and Honeydew Melon Salad (page 297) with ½ cup of your favorite fruit yogurt
Snacks	• Choose 3 separate snacks from the MediterrAsian-Friendly Snacks list on page 126, and enjoy them throughout the day between meals.
Beverages	• 1 to 2 cups of tea or coffee • 1 to 2 glasses of wine or beer • A glass of freshly squeezed juice • Plenty of water
Natural Movement	• Be physically active for at least 20 minutes. Choose from the Natural Movement ideas on page 68, or come up with your own.
Calm Time	• Physically and emotionally relax for at least 30 minutes. Choose from the Calm Time ideas on page 87, or come up with your own.

Piece of fruit (such as an orange, apple, pear, or peach)

Small bowl of fresh fruit salad topped with a little fruit yogurt

Handful of berries like strawberries or raspberries

Wedge of melon

Small bunch of grapes

Handful of cherries

Small fruit platter

Sliced apple or pear with a little thinly sliced Parmesan cheese

Mashed banana spread on a slice of whole-grain bread or a whole-grain cracker and dusted lightly with cinnamon

½ cup fruit yogurt sprinkled with crushed nuts

Handful of dried figs and pistachios

Handful of dried dates and walnuts

Handful of dried apricots and cashew nuts

Handful of nuts (such as walnuts, almonds, cashews, peanuts, pistachios, and macadamias)

Handful of slivered or flaked almonds and raisins

Handful of toasted sunflower seeds

Handful of pecans served with a little blue cheese (like gorgonzola)

Handful of trail mix

Whole-grain cracker topped with a little thinly sliced sharp cheese, sliced tomato, sea salt, and freshly ground black pepper

Whole-grain cracker topped with smoked salmon, capers, dill, sea salt, freshly ground black pepper, and drizzled with lemon juice

Whole-grain cracker topped with 1 tablespoon of Savory Salmon Spread (page 290) or Savory Tuna Spread (page 290)

Whole-grain cracker topped with ricotta cheese and sun-dried tomatoes

Whole-grain cracker topped with a little goat cheese and sliced stuffed green olives

Slice of whole-grain bread or toast topped with a tablespoon of natural peanut butter

Piece of bruschetta spread lightly with pesto

Half dozen cherry tomatoes with 1 ounce (30 g) of cubed cheddar cheese

6 olives and a little thinly sliced sharp cheese

3 jarred marinated bell pepper strips with a little finely sliced Parmesan cheese

6 canned smoked oysters

Half a small can of baby shrimp, wrapped in a lettuce leaf with half a sliced tomato and a teaspoon of mayonnaise

Half a small can of tuna with sliced tomato and 4 olives

Handful of pita wedges dipped in a little hummus

Vegetable crudités served with a little hummus

2 dolmades (stuffed grape leaves)

Handful of pretzels

Cup of air-popped popcorn (popcorn is a whole grain!)

Boiled egg lightly sprinkled with sea salt

⅓ cup cold baked beans

Small bowl of your favorite whole-grain breakfast cereal

½ ounce (15 g) high-quality dark chocolate

Living the MediterrAsian Way: Eleven Lifestyle Scenarios

Here are eleven lifestyle scenarios that show you how a MediterrAsian way of living can easily be adapted and customized to fit into any lifestyle and any situation. These scenarios also highlight how fun, easy, and flexible it is to follow a MediterrAsian way of living on a day-to-day basis.

Relaxing Weekend at Home

Morning

BREAKFAST: For a breakfast with an Italian twist this morning, make Italian-Style Scrambled Eggs (page 264). Enjoy a good strong cup of coffee, and finish with a bowl of grapes topped with a dollop of fruit yogurt.

CALM TIME: Visit the library and browse for books. The quiet serenity of the library is a real break from noise pollution. Look for some interesting cookbooks based on Mediterranean and Asian cuisine for recipe ideas.

SNACK: 3 dried figs make the perfect chewy sweet treat.

Afternoon

LUNCH: Enjoy the beautiful weather by having an outdoor barbecue for lunch. Instead of the usual grilled beef steak and sausages, opt for grilled salmon steak and tender grilled shrimp. Serve this with a crusty whole-grain roll and mixed salad leaves drizzled with a little extra-virgin olive oil and balsamic vinegar. And what better way to wash down a hot barbecue than with a glass of icy cold beer. Finish the barbecue with some fresh sliced melon.

NATURAL MOVEMENT: After lunch has had a little time to go down, head to the local park with a friend and play Frisbee.

SNACK: A handful of creamy macadamia nuts will keep hunger at bay until dinner.

Evening

DINNER AND DESSERT: For something quick and tasty, cook up a Fragrant Chicken and Vegetable Stir-Fry (page 158). Follow this with some sliced kiwi fruit and banana topped with a scoop of favorite ice cream.

NATURAL MOVEMENT: Before it gets dark, walk the dog and check out the beautiful sunset on the way home.

SNACK: A handful of pretzels.

CALM TIME: Dust off your old photo albums and have a nostalgic look through your past.

Hectic Weekend at Home

Morning

BREAKFAST: A Sardine Toast Topper (page 265) served with fresh juice and followed by some crisp sliced apple will make the perfect energy-filled start to the day.

NATURAL MOVEMENT: The first jobs of the day are to mow the lawn and get rid of some of those weeds that have accumulated in the backyard.

SNACK: Gardening is hungry work, so grab a handful of almonds and enjoy a refreshing mango.

Afternoon

NATURAL MOVEMENT: As part of your hectic day you have to do some shopping at the mall. As you drive into the parking lot you see dozens of people circling around trying to find the closest spot. Simply park at the far end of the lot and walk the extra distance. The people who are circling the mall look on jealously as you enter the mall before them.

LUNCH: At the mall pop into a sandwich shop and have them assemble a big MediterrAsian-balanced sandwich with roast chicken, peppers, tomatoes, pickles, lettuce, olives, mustard, and a little mayo on whole-grain bread.

CALM TIME AND NATURAL MOVEMENT: After lunch, take ten minutes for yourself and window-shop at your favorite stores.

SNACK: A juicy mandarin not only makes a sweet snack, but it also quenches your thirst after all that exhausting window-shopping.

Evening

DINNER AND DESSERT: Take a break from cooking tonight, and order in a MediterrAsian-balanced meal from the local Chinese restaurant instead. Wash it down with a cold beer. For dessert, carry on the Asian theme and have a fortune cookie, then some canned lychees and pineapple in natural juice with a scoop of your favorite ice cream.

SNACK: A couple of thin slices of sharp cheddar cheese and half a dozen olives.

CALM TIME: About 20 minutes before bedtime, find a quite place in the house by yourself, light a candle and incense, put on some soft music, and meditate. This not only calms your mind and helps you reconnect with your spirit, it also sets you up for an extra-sound sleep.

Morning

BREAKFAST: Today is a busy day—deadlines are backing up and time is scarce. But it is important to be mentally focused for the busy day ahead, so quickly have a bowl of muesli topped with sliced kiwi fruit.

NATURAL MOVEMENT: You can't afford to get stuck in traffic and be late for work, so catch the bus instead. The five-minute walk to the bus stop isn't only a good opportunity for some natural movement, it also provides a chance to gather your thoughts for the day ahead. At work, instead of taking the elevator, simply walk up the four flights of stairs.

SNACK: Midmorning, enjoy two biscotti and a cup of coffee.

Afternoon

LUNCH: Lunchtime and there's no time to lose. You need to keep your energy up and your hunger at bay—but there's only a short time for lunch, so pop into a Lebanese takeout and grab a pita bread stuffed with falafel, salad, and hummus and drizzled with a little chili sauce. While still out and about, pop into the deli and grab a handful of succulent cherries for a sweet finish.

CALM TIME: On the way back to work, stop at the park for five minutes and take in the fresh air, the sounds of the birds singing, and the wonderful colors of nature.

SNACK: It's midafternoon and time to satisfy an attack of the munchies. A handful of cashew nuts and a dozen grapes soon fix that problem.

NATURAL MOVEMENT: Walk from work to the bus stop; then at the other end, walk from the local bus stop home.

Evening

DINNER AND DESSERT: Arriving home exhausted, you simply order in a MediterrAsian-friendly pizza. To accompany the meal, have a glass of red wine, and for dessert enjoy some sliced strawberries topped with ½ cup of your favorite fruit yogurt.

CALM TIME: It's been a taxing day. After dinner fill a large bowl with hot water, add a few drops of aromatherapy oil, and soak your feet for 20 minutes.

SNACK: A whole-grain cracker topped with some thinly sliced cheese, sliced tomato, and a little freshly ground pepper and sea salt.

Relaxed Work Day

Morning

BREAKFAST: For something hot and sweet this morning, make a bowl of Creamy Fruit and Nut Oatmeal (page 266) and accompany it with a cup of coffee.

SNACK: A handful of mixed nuts and a glass of fresh juice satisfy the midmorning munchies.

Afternoon

LUNCH: Take a little extra time in the morning to make a Curried Egg and Salad Sandwich (page 120), and keep it in the staff refrigerator to enjoy at lunch. Follow this with 6 fresh strawberries.

NATURAL MOVEMENT: Instead of talking to colleagues on the phone or via e-mail, walk up and down the stairs to talk to them. Not only does this slip in some natural movement, but it's nice to have the extra bit of human contact.

CALM TIME: At lunch, pop into a day spa close to work and have a rejuvenating 20-minute neck and shoulder massage.

SNACK: Treat yourself to 2 squares of good-quality dark chocolate.

Evening

NATURAL MOVEMENT: Straight after work, meet up with a friend and play a bit of tennis at your local sports club.

DINNER AND DESSERT: Quickly whip up some Pasta with Arugula, Fava Beans, and Prosciutto (page 151), and serve it with a simple green salad and a glass of red wine. For dessert have a slice of fruit cake.

SNACK: A cup of air-popped popcorn.

CALM TIME: Snuggle up in bed with your favorite book and slowly drift off to sleep.

Weekday with the Kids

Morning

BREAKFAST: It's got to be something quick and nourishing this morning, so enjoy a bowl of Raisin, Apricot, and Almond Muesli (page 266).

NATURAL MOVEMENT: Walk to the bus stop to see your older kids off to school. Take along the youngest in a stroller, which adds intensity to the walk.

SNACK: While out and about, pop into the store and pick up a small bag of jellybeans.

Afternoon

NATURAL MOVEMENT: There's lots of energetic cleaning and tidying around the house to be done, including making beds, picking up toys, hanging out the washing, and vacuuming the floors.

LUNCH: For lunch thaw some frozen precooked shrimp in hot water for five minutes and make up a shrimp and salad sandwich on whole-grain bread. For a sweet finish, have three fresh, juicy plums.

CALM TIME AND NATURAL MOVEMENT: With the chores out of the way, it gives you a good opportunity to have a relaxing play with the little one.

SNACK: A slice of whole-grain bread spread with natural peanut butter.

Evening

DINNER AND DESSERT: Use that premade fresh pesto purchased from the deli this morning when you walked the kids to the bus stop to quickly make Pesto Pasta with Salmon, Broccoli, and Roasted Red Pepper (page 149). Accompany this with a glass of red wine. For dessert enjoy some Mango, Grape, and Honeydew Melon Salad (page 297) served with a scoop of gelato.

CALM TIME: While your other half looks after the kids, pop away into the bedroom, open up your soul, and write down your thoughts, feelings, and observations in a private journal.

SNACK: Over a favorite TV show, enjoy a handful of pistachio nuts and 4 dried dates.

Weekend with the Kids

Morning

BREAKFAST: For a quick, hearty, and healthy breakfast that everyone will enjoy, make up some baked beans on whole-grain toast. Wash this down with a cold glass of orange juice and finish off with a fresh peach.

NATURAL MOVEMENT: The car is looking pretty grubby, and the kids are looking bored—what a great opportunity to fix both problems at once and clean the car together! Not only will the car end up clean and shiny, but you'll also have lots of fun getting wet and having water fights in the process.

SNACK: A small piece of lightly buttered fruit cake with a cup of tea is just what's needed to see you through to lunchtime.

Afternoon

LUNCH: For lunch, keep the kids happy by making burgers (page 225) and oven-baked fries, but get the kids involved in the preparation and cooking. This isn't only a good bonding experience—it also cuts cooking time in half! After lunch enjoy ½ cup of strawberry yogurt.

NATURAL MOVEMENT: After lunch take the kids to the local zoo and have a good walk, checking out all the different animals.

SNACK: A handful of cashews will satisfy your hunger and help keep energy levels up.

CALM TIME: Late afternoon call up a close friend and have a relaxing chat.

Evening

DINNER AND DESSERT: Make a Sicilian Tuna and Basil Pizza (page 169), and wash it down with a glass of red wine. For dessert have something fun and colorful—chunks of papaya and pineapple topped with yogurt and passion fruit.

CALM TIME: After dinner surf the net with the kids.

SNACK: A handful of Brazil nuts.

Dinner Party

Morning

BREAKFAST: Dinner guests will be arriving at 7:30 P.M., and the predinner party jitters make the thought of eating a big breakfast unappealing. But you need plenty of energy for the day ahead, so have a small bowl of favorite whole-grain cereal topped with sliced strawberries.

NATURAL MOVEMENT: The place needs a good dust and tidy up before the guests arrive so pop on your cleaning clothes and set to work transforming your house through a "cardio-cleaning blitz."

SNACK: Relax for 10 minutes and have a biscotti with a cup of coffee.

Afternoon

LUNCH: Whip up a tuna sandwich with lettuce and tomato on multigrain bread, then finish with a juicy nectarine.

NATURAL MOVEMENT: Time to grab some last-minute fresh ingredients from the local store. Instead of spending time warming up the car, opening and closing the garage door, and having to find a parking spot at the other end, walk instead (it's nice to get some fresh air after being stuck in the house all morning). At the store, pick up a copy of your favorite magazine.

CALM TIME: After finishing the cleaning and other chores, there's still plenty of time before you need to start preparing for the night ahead. So slip away into the peace and calm of the bedroom and have a 20-minute browse through the magazine you picked up at the store.

SNACK: A handful of almonds and a small bunch of grapes boost energy for the dinner preparation and help to keep you mentally focused for the night ahead.

Evening

DINNER AND DESSERT: All week you've been thinking about what food to serve at the dinner party. Opt for a Mediterranean theme—Greek—and serve Greek Shrimp with Feta (page 179) and Greek Salad (page 253) with fresh crusty bread. For dessert it has to be something sweet and yummy, so try Mixed Berry Coulis with Greek Vanilla Yogurt (page 292).

Everyone at the dinner party thinks you've been slaving away in the kitchen all day, but little do they know it's taken only a little more than an hour to prepare and cook the lot. And no one can believe that the decadent and delicious food they're eating is also incredibly good for them.

SNACK: Too full from dinner to even contemplate having something to eat? Instead, have a soothing cup of antioxidant-rich tea.

CALM TIME: It's been a tiring but ultimately very exhilarating day. Reflect on the successful night while having a long, hot, calming soak in the shower.

Romantic Weekend

Morning

BREAKFAST: For a special breakfast for you and your loved one, prepare scrambled eggs with smoked salmon on whole-grain English muffins. Accompany this with coffee and juice.

CALM TIME: Relax into the morning by reading the local weekend paper, paying particular interest to the food, social, travel, and living sections.

SNACK: A crunchy sliced apple and a little thinly sliced Parmesan cheese.

Afternoon

LUNCH: Go for a long drive to somewhere scenic and relaxing, and find a pretty, grassy area and set up a picnic blanket. For your romantic picnic have an Italian-Style Chicken Sandwich with Pesto-Mayonnaise (page 232) and a selection of sliced cheeses, crackers, and fresh and dried fruit, all washed down with a bubbly glass of champagne.

NATURAL MOVEMENT: After lunch make the most of the wonderful outdoors and go for a scenic walk.

SNACK: A handful of cashew nuts will help get you through to dinner.

Evening

DINNER AND DESSERT: To carry on the romance of the day, go to a restaurant for dinner. The Italian place up the road serves salmon risotto to die for. On the side have some crusty bread drizzled with a little extra-virgin olive oil, and wash it all down with a glass of red wine. For dessert have something special and order tiramisu (a luxurious dessert made with coffee- and chocolate-infused sponge cakes and mascarpone cheese) accompanied with fresh sliced melon.

CALM TIME AND SNACK: After returning home from dinner, light a couple of candles and a stick of incense, have a nice long soak in the bath with your partner, and feed each other grapes.

NATURAL MOVEMENT: After the bath, retire to the bedroom to do what comes naturally!

Party Night

Morning

BREAKFAST: There's a big party tonight, but all you can think about right now is how hungry you are for a substantial and savory breakfast. So make an Italian-Style Pan-Fried Sandwich (page 268), and wash it down with a cup of coffee. Afterward, have 3 juicy plums.

CALM TIME: Sink back in a comfy chair and have a relaxing read for 20 minutes.

SNACK: A handful of almonds.

NATURAL MOVEMENT: Because there might be some dancing at the party tonight, get in a little practice—pop on your favorite CD and dance around the house.

Afternoon

LUNCH: For lunch heat up a bowl of Minestrone Soup (page 240), frozen from when you made it a fortnight ago. Finish with a sliced banana topped with a dollop of fruit yogurt.

CALM TIME: To relax your body and calm your mind before the party tonight, put on some loose and comfortable clothes, lay a towel down on the floor, and practice yoga for 20 minutes.

SNACK: A handful of pretzels.

Evening

DINNER AND DESSERT: There are going to be lots of snacks at the party, so have a relatively light dinner and put together a Salade Niçoise (page 254) with a little crusty whole-grain bread on the side. For dessert opt for something easy and simply have an orange.

SNACK: For the party bring along a selection of vegetable crudités accompanied with homemade hummus (page 284) for dipping. You end up going a little overboard on your alcohol intake, but that's fine because parties only happen occasionally, and besides you'll be back to your healthy moderate drinking habits tomorrow.

NATURAL MOVEMENT: Good thing you practiced your dance moves earlier today, because as the night wears on and everyone gets more and more relaxed, the evening turns into a dance party!

At 30,000 Feet

Morning

BREAKFAST: You're going on a long flight later today, and you realize you'll need lots of energy for packing your bags and lugging them around, so start the day with a generous bowl of Raisin, Apricot, and Almond Muesli (page 266).

CALM TIME: It's a lovely sunny morning, so go out into the backyard, stand under the dappled shade of a tree, and relax your mind and body by practicing tai chi.

SNACK: 2 succulent fresh apricots.

NATURAL MOVEMENT: Pack your bags and carry them out to the car.

Afternoon

LUNCH: Don't eat anything too rich before the flight. Luckily there's a Japanese restaurant close to the airport that serves great lunches; so stop in and have a warming bowl of miso soup, a selection of fresh tuna, salmon, and shrimp sushi, and finish with a bowl of fresh fruit salad.

NATURAL MOVEMENT: When you arrive at the airport, carry your bags up to the counter. After you've checked your luggage, have a good walk around the airport checking out the duty-free stores.

SNACK: It's more than an hour until your flight, so grab a small chocolate bar from a newsstand.

Evening

DINNER AND DESSERT: You made sure to request a seafood meal for the flight. Luckily, this means you get your meal before everyone else, and your meal also is healthier and just as tasty. Accompany your meal with a glass of wine.

CALM TIME: Completely relax and make the most of the entertainment on the plane including movies, magazines, and audio broadcasts.

SNACK: Buzz a flight attendant and ask for a package of pretzels and another glass of wine.

On Vacation

Morning

BREAKFAST: After a sleep-in, enjoy breakfast at a local café. Order a smoked salmon bagel (spread thinly with cream cheese and topped with dill and capers), some grilled tomatoes, and a cappuccino. Finish with a refreshing fruit salad with a dollop of yogurt.

NATURAL MOVEMENT AND CALM TIME: What better way to familiarize yourself with a new place than a bit of sightseeing. You've thought ahead and already booked a guided walking tour. While on the tour, take lots of photos to capture the memories forever.

SNACK: A handful of sweet and chewy dates.

Afternoon

LUNCH: For something quick and familiar, grab lunch from a burger bar. Instead of going straight for the beef burger with cheese, order something equally tasty but more MediterrAsian-balanced: a grilled chicken burger with lots of salad veggies, including lettuce, tomatoes, onions, and pickles. Finish with a juicy pear.

CALM TIME AND NATURAL MOVEMENT: There are so many new stores to discover and souvenirs to be collected, so go on a relaxing shopping spree.

SNACK: A handful of macadamia nuts and a dozen grapes will provide even more energy for sightseeing and shopping.

Evening

DINNER AND DESSERT: There is no shortage of Chinese, Italian, and Indian restaurants nearby. Opt for Indian food and enjoy a spicy shrimp and almond curry served over basmati rice with a vegetable side dish and naan bread. Wash it all down with a glass of cold beer.

CALM TIME: Back at the hotel, relax into the night by watching a funny video.

SNACK: A small bag of baked corn chips makes a great accompaniment to the video.

Recipes

Pasta Dishes

Pasta Puttanesca

This robust pasta dish originated in Naples, named after the local women of easy virtue. All the ingredients are just as easy to put your hands on, making this a quick and satisfying meal!

SERVES 4

6 tablespoons extra-virgin olive oil
2 onions, finely chopped
4 cloves garlic, finely chopped
8 anchovy fillets, chopped
2 small red chiles, deseeded and finely chopped
4 teaspoons capers, rinsed and drained
16 pitted black olives, quartered
28 ounces (840 g) canned tomatoes, chopped
1 teaspoon sea salt
½ teaspoon freshly ground black pepper
1 pound (500 g) spaghetti
2 tablespoons finely chopped fresh flat-leaf parsley

Bring a large pot of water to a boil.

Heat 4 tablespoons of the oil in a skillet over medium heat and cook the onions for 6 minutes, stirring occasionally. Add the garlic and anchovies and cook for 1 minute, stirring to break up the anchovies. Add the chiles, capers, olives, tomatoes, salt, and pepper, and bring to a boil. Reduce the heat to medium-low and simmer, uncovered, for 10 minutes, stirring occasionally.

While the sauce is simmering, add the pasta to the boiling water and cook according to package directions. Drain the cooked pasta in a colander and put the sauce in the bottom of the empty pot. Top with the hot pasta, parsley, and reserved 2 tablespoons of olive oil, and toss together gently to combine.

VARIATION: For a more protein-packed meal, add a 12-ounce (360 g) can of tuna (drained and flaked) to the sauce at the end of cooking to heat through.

Pasta Primavera

A vegetable-packed pasta dish with asparagus, cherry tomatoes, mushrooms, peas, and green beans, combined with toasted pine nuts and topped with Parmesan cheese.

SERVES 4

4 tablespoons pine nuts
1 pound (500 g) dried pasta of your choice (penne works well)
6 tablespoons extra-virgin olive oil
2 red onions, finely chopped
4 cloves garlic, finely chopped
20 cherry tomatoes, halved
16 fresh asparagus spears, bottoms trimmed, cut into 2-inch pieces
24 green beans, ends trimmed, halved
1 cup frozen green peas, thawed
8 button mushrooms, sliced
4 tablespoons finely chopped fresh basil
½ cup white wine
2 teaspoons sea salt
1 teaspoon freshly ground black pepper
Grated Parmesan cheese

Heat a skillet over medium heat; add the pine nuts and toast, stirring continuously, for 1 minute; set aside.

Bring a large pot of water to a boil. Add the pasta and cook according to package directions.

While the pasta is cooking, heat 4 tablespoons of the olive oil in a large skillet over medium heat and cook the onions, stirring, for 6 minutes. Add the garlic and cook for another minute. Add the tomatoes, asparagus, and green beans and cook, stirring regularly, for 2 minutes. Add the peas, mushrooms, basil, wine, salt, and pepper; cover the skillet and cook for 5 minutes. Add the remaining 2 tablespoons of olive oil and the toasted pine nuts, and stir to combine all the ingredients.

Drain the cooked pasta in a colander, and put the vegetable mixture in the bottom of the empty pot. Top with the hot pasta and toss together gently to combine well and heat through. Serve the pasta topped with a little Parmesan cheese.

VARIATION: Substitute some or all of the vegetables with broccoli, carrots, zucchini, or fresh corn kernels.

Lemony Tuna, Olive, and Vegetable Pasta

This pasta dish is extraordinarily easy to prepare and absolutely delicious to eat. Simply mix the ingredients together in a bowl while the pasta, beans, and red bell peppers cook in the same pot of boiling water. Put the uncooked sauce in the pasta pot and toss with the hot, drained pasta and vegetables to heat through.

SERVES 4

1 pound (500 g) pasta of your choice (fusilli works well)

24 green beans, ends trimmed and halved

2 red bell peppers, julienned

12 ounces (360 g) canned light tuna in olive oil, drained and broken into chunks

6 tablespoons extra-virgin olive oil

4 tablespoons freshly squeezed lemon juice

16 pitted black olives, sliced

2 tablespoons chopped fresh flat-leaf parsley

2 tablespoons capers, rinsed, drained, and chopped

2 cloves garlic, minced

1 teaspoon freshly grated lemon zest

1 teaspoon sea salt

½ teaspoon freshly ground black pepper

Bring a large pot of water to a boil. Add the pasta and cook according to package directions, adding the green beans and bell peppers to the pot for the final 8 minutes of cooking.

While the pasta is cooking, in a small bowl, mix together the tuna, olive oil, lemon juice, olives, parsley, capers, garlic, lemon zest, salt, and pepper. Drain the cooked pasta and vegetables in a colander, then put the tuna mixture in the bottom of the empty pot and top with the hot pasta and vegetables. Toss together gently to combine well and heat through.

VARIATION: Toss 4 cups of broccoli florets into the boiling pasta water instead of the green beans. Serve with a little grated Parmesan or Romano cheese if desired.

Pasta with Shrimp and Chile

This simple recipe combines shrimp, chiles, and tomatoes with white wine to make a spicy sauce to toss with your favorite pasta.

4 tablespoons extra-virgin olive oil
2 green bell peppers, julienned
4 cloves garlic, finely chopped
4 small red chiles, deseeded and finely chopped
28 ounces (840 g) canned tomatoes, chopped
1 cup white wine
1 pound (500 g) dried pasta of your choice (spaghetti or fettuccine works well)
32 large uncooked shrimp (prawns), peeled
2 teaspoons sea salt
1 teaspoon freshly ground black pepper
2 tablespoons freshly squeezed lemon juice
2 tablespoons finely chopped fresh flat-leaf parsley

Bring a large pot of water to a boil.

Heat the olive oil in a skillet over medium heat and cook the bell pepper, stirring occasionally, for 6 minutes. Add the garlic and chiles and cook for another minute. Add the tomatoes and white wine and simmer for 10 minutes.

While the sauce simmers, add the pasta to the boiling water and cook according to package directions.

Add the shrimp, salt, and pepper to the sauce and simmer, covered, for 5 minutes more, then stir in the lemon juice and parsley. Drain the cooked pasta into a colander and put the tomato-shrimp sauce in the bottom of the empty pot. Top with the hot pasta and toss together gently to combine well.

VARIATION: Use scallops instead of shrimp, or replace the wine with good-quality fish stock.

Sicilian Pasta with Broccoli, Raisins, and Pine Nuts

This traditional Sicilian pasta dish combines the saltiness of anchovies with the sweetness of raisins.

SERVES 4

4 tablespoons pine nuts
4 tablespoons extra-virgin olive oil
2 onions, finely chopped
2 cloves garlic, finely chopped
8 anchovy fillets, chopped
2 cups canned whole tomatoes, chopped
2 tablespoons tomato paste
4 tablespoons raisins, soaked in ½ cup of hot water while you prepare
   the other ingredients
1 teaspoon sea salt
½ teaspoon freshly ground black pepper
1 pound (500 g) pasta of your choice (farfalle or penne works well)
4 cups broccoli florets
8 tablespoons grated Parmesan or Romano cheese

Toast the pine nuts in a skillet over medium heat for 1 minute; set aside. Bring a large pot of water to a boil.

Heat the olive oil in a skillet over medium heat and cook the onions, stirring occasionally, for 6 minutes. Add the garlic and anchovies and cook, stirring to break up the anchovies, for 1 minute. Add the tomatoes, tomato paste, raisins and their soaking water, salt, and pepper. Bring to a boil, cover with a lid, reduce the heat to low, and simmer gently for 10 minutes.

While the sauce simmers, add the pasta to the boiling water and cook according to package directions, adding the broccoli to the pot for the final 6 minutes of cooking. Drain the cooked pasta and broccoli in a colander and put the sauce in the bottom of the empty pot. Top with the hot pasta, broccoli, and toasted pine nuts, and toss together gently to combine well. Serve the pasta sprinkled with the Parmesan cheese.

Pesto Pasta with Salmon, Broccoli, and Roasted Red Pepper

This dish takes very little time to prepare and cook, yet it's packed with flavor and nutrients. A fresh green salad makes the perfect accompaniment.

SERVES 4

1 pound (500 g) pasta of your choice (penne or fusilli works well)
24 ounces (720 g) uncooked salmon fillet, cut into bite-size pieces
4 cups broccoli florets
½ cup jarred roasted red bell peppers, roughly chopped
1½ cups pesto sauce, homemade (page 278) or store-bought

Bring a large pot of water to a boil. Add the pasta and cook according to package directions, adding the salmon and broccoli to the pot for the final 6 minutes of cooking. Drain the cooked pasta, salmon, and broccoli in a colander, reserving 4 tablespoons of the cooking water in the pot. Put the bell peppers and pesto in the bottom of the pot and top with the hot pasta, salmon, and broccoli. Toss together gently to combine well and heat through.

VARIATION: Replace the salmon with bite-size pieces of chicken breast.

Sublime Seafood Pasta

In this mouthwatering dish, a selection of fresh and succulent seafood is cooked in a tomato, garlic, basil, and olive oil sauce, then tossed with hot pasta.

SERVES 4

4 tablespoons extra-virgin olive oil
2 onions, finely chopped
2 zucchini, sliced into ½-inch rounds
4 cloves garlic, finely chopped
28 ounces (840 g) canned tomatoes, chopped
1 cup white wine
2 tablespoons tomato paste
2 teaspoons sea salt
1 teaspoon freshly ground black pepper
1 pound (500 g) pasta of your choice (conchiglie or fusilli works well)
12 ounces (360 g) uncooked salmon fillet, cut into bite-size pieces
16 large uncooked shrimp (prawns), peeled
16 uncooked large scallops
4 tablespoons finely chopped fresh basil
2 tablespoons freshly squeezed lemon juice

Bring a large pot of water to a boil.

Heat the oil in a large skillet over medium heat and cook the onions, stirring occasionally, for 6 minutes. Add the zucchini and garlic and cook, stirring, for 2 minutes. Add the tomatoes, wine, tomato paste, salt, and pepper and simmer for 10 minutes.

While the sauce simmers, add the pasta to the boiling water and cook according to package directions.

Add the salmon, shrimp, scallops, and basil to the sauce, simmer, covered, for 6 minutes, then stir in the lemon juice. Drain the cooked pasta in a colander and put the tomato-seafood sauce in the bottom of the empty pot. Top with the hot pasta and toss together gently to combine well.

TIP: Look at the selection available at the seafood counter and base your choices on what looks freshest and best, or buy a frozen seafood mix, which usually contains a blend that may include shrimp, squid, mussels, and fish.

Pasta with Arugula, Fava Beans, and Prosciutto

This pasta dish uses meat in a traditionally Mediterranean way: in small amounts as a flavor and texture enhancer.

SERVES 4

1 pound (500 g) pasta of your choice (penne works well)
2 cups frozen fava (broad) beans, thawed, leathery outer skin removed
4 cups arugula (rocket), stems trimmed, leaves washed, and roughly chopped
4 tablespoons extra-virgin olive oil
7 ounces (200 g) thinly sliced prosciutto, chopped
4 cloves garlic, finely chopped
20 pitted black olives, halved
4 tablespoons chopped fresh flat-leaf parsley
1 teaspoon sea salt
½ teaspoon freshly ground black pepper
8 tablespoons grated Parmesan or Romano cheese

Bring a large pot of water to a boil. Add the pasta to the boiling water and cook according to package directions, adding the fava beans and arugula to the pot for the final 2 minutes of cooking.

While the pasta is cooking, heat the oil in a skillet over medium heat and cook the prosciutto and garlic, stirring occasionally, for 2 minutes. Drain the cooked pasta, fava beans, and arugula in a colander, reserving 4 tablespoons of cooking water in the pot. Put the garlic and prosciutto in the bottom of the pot, and top with the hot pasta, fava beans, and arugula. Add the olives, parsley, salt, and pepper, and toss together gently to combine well and heat through. Serve the pasta sprinkled with the Parmesan or Romano cheese.

Pasta with Salsa Verde and Smoked Salmon

Salsa verde, a classic Italian green sauce, is simply wonderful tossed with smoked salmon and pasta. The anchovies and smoked salmon in this recipe are good sources of healthy omega-3 fatty acids, and are handy alternatives to fresh fish.

SERVES 4

1 pound (500 g) pasta of your choice (spaghetti or fettuccine works well)
2 zucchini, cut into ¼-inch rounds
⅔ cup Salsa Verde (page 285)
7 ounces (200 g) sliced smoked salmon, cut into thin strips

Bring a large pot of water to a boil. Add the pasta to the boiling water and cook according to package directions, adding the zucchini to the pot for the final 5 minutes of cooking.

Drain the cooked pasta and zucchini in a colander, reserving 4 tablespoons of cooking water in the pot. Put the salsa verde and salmon in the bottom of the pot and top with the hot pasta and zucchini. Toss together gently to combine well and heat through.

VARIATION: Use strips of cooked skinless chicken breast in place of the smoked salmon.

Creamy Chicken, Mushroom, and Sun-Dried Tomato Pasta

A delightfully creamy pasta dish dotted with bite-size pieces of chicken and sliced mushrooms and sun-dried tomatoes. Scallions are also known as spring onions.

SERVES 4

1 pound (500 g) pasta (farfalle or penne works well)
24 ounces (720 g) boneless skinless chicken breasts, cut into bite-size pieces
2 cups broccoli florets
4 tablespoons extra-virgin olive oil
2 cups sliced button mushrooms
6 tablespoons finely chopped sun-dried tomatoes in oil
4 scallions (white and green parts), trimmed and thinly sliced
4 cloves garlic, finely chopped
2 cups fish, vegetable, or chicken stock
2 cups milk
6 tablespoons cornstarch (corn flour), mixed to a paste with 6 tablespoons water
1⅓ cups grated Parmesan cheese
1 teaspoon sea salt
½ teaspoon freshly ground black pepper

Bring a large pot of water to a boil. Add the pasta to the boiling water and cook according to package directions, adding the chicken to the pot for the final 8 minutes of cooking and the broccoli for the final 6 minutes of cooking.

While the pasta is cooking, heat the oil in a skillet over medium heat and cook the mushrooms, sun-dried tomatoes, scallions, and garlic, stirring occasionally, for 3 minutes. Add the stock and milk and heat until almost boiling. Stir the cornstarch mixture into the hot milk and stock in the skillet, continue stirring until thickened. Stir in the Parmesan cheese, salt, and pepper until well combined.

Drain the pasta, chicken, and broccoli in a colander. Put the creamy sauce in the bottom of the empty pot, top with the hot pasta, chicken, and broccoli, then toss together gently to combine well.

Pasta with Tuna, Green Beans, Olives, and Romesco Sauce

Freshly cooked pasta and green beans are tossed with chunks of tuna, olives, and a robust sauce made with roasted red peppers and toasted almonds for a pasta dish with a Spanish twist.

SERVES 4

1 pound (500 g) pasta of your choice (fusilli or penne works well)
32 green beans, ends trimmed, cut in half
2 cups Romesco Sauce (page 283)
12 ounces (360 g) canned light meat tuna in olive oil, drained
    and broken into chunks
24 pitted black olives, halved

Bring a large pot of water to a boil. Add the pasta to the boiling water and cook according to package directions, adding the green beans to the pot for the final 6 minutes of cooking. Drain the cooked pasta and green beans in a colander, reserving 4 tablespoons of cooking water in the pot. Put the Romesco Sauce in the bottom of the pot and top with the hot pasta, tuna, green beans, and olives. Toss together gently to combine well and heat through.

VARIATION: This dish is also delicious with broccoli instead of green beans.

Stir-Fries

Stir-Fried Scallops and Vegetables with Honey-Ginger Sauce

Succulent scallops are stir-fried with aromatic ginger and fresh vegetables, then glazed with a Chinese honey-ginger sauce.

SERVES 4

2 cups long-grain white rice
4 tablespoons soy sauce
4 tablespoons oyster sauce
2 tablespoons Chinese rice wine (or dry sherry)
4 teaspoons honey
4 tablespoons peanut or canola oil
24 uncooked large scallops
2 carrots, peeled and julienned
2 green bell peppers, julienned
2 zucchini (courgettes), sliced into ¼-inch rounds
4 cloves garlic, minced
4 teaspoons finely grated fresh ginger
2 cups fish, chicken, or vegetable stock
2 tablespoons cornstarch (corn flour), mixed to a paste with 2 tablespoons water
2 scallions (white and green parts), trimmed and thinly sliced

Bring 3 cups of water to a boil in a saucepan. Stir in the rice, and keep stirring until the water returns to a boil. Cover the pot with a tight-fitting lid, reduce the heat to very low, and simmer gently for 15 minutes.

While the rice cooks, mix together the soy sauce, oyster sauce, Chinese rice wine, and honey in a bowl. Heat a wok or large skillet over high heat, add 2 tablespoons of the oil, and cook the scallops until cooked through, about 1½ minutes, turning once while cooking. Remove the scallops from the wok and set aside on a plate.

Heat the remaining oil in the wok and stir-fry the carrots and bell peppers for 3 minutes. Add the zucchini and stir-fry for another 2 minutes. Add the garlic and ginger and stir-fry for 1 minute, then return the scallops to the wok. Add the sauce mixture and stock. Add the cornstarch paste and cook until thickened and thoroughly combined, then toss with the scallions. Serve on a bed of the rice.

VARIATION: Use chicken or shrimp instead of scallops.

Stir-Fried Tofu, Vegetables, and Water Chestnuts in Oyster Sauce

This stir-fry features tofu, assorted vegetables, and crunchy water chestnuts in a thick Chinese oyster sauce.

SERVES 4

8 ounces (240 g) dried wheat noodles
6 tablespoons oyster sauce
4 tablespoons soy sauce
4 tablespoons water
4 tablespoons of peanut or canola oil
30 green beans, ends trimmed, halved
2 red bell peppers, julienned
12 ounces (360 g) firm tofu, cut into small cubes
1 cup canned water chestnuts, rinsed and drained
2 scallions (white and green parts), trimmed and thinly sliced
4 cloves garlic, minced
4 teaspoons finely grated fresh ginger

Add the dried noodles to a saucepan of boiling water and cook for 5 minutes.

While the noodles cook, mix together the oyster sauce, soy sauce, and water in a small bowl. Heat a wok or large skillet over high heat; add the oil and stir-fry the beans for 2 minutes. Add the bell peppers and stir-fry for 2 minutes. Add the tofu and stir-fry for 3 minutes. Add the water chestnuts, scallions, garlic, and ginger and stir-fry for 1 minute. Add the sauce mixture and mix to heat through. Serve on a bed of the noodles.

Fragrant Chicken and Vegetable Stir-Fry

A combination of colorful, crunchy vegetables are stir-fried with pieces of tender chicken and tossed in a rich, aromatic sauce.

SERVES 4

8 ounces (240 g) dried wheat noodles
4 tablespoons soy sauce
4 tablespoons oyster sauce
2 tablespoons Chinese rice wine (or dry sherry)
1 tablespoon sesame oil
1 teaspoon five-spice powder
1 tablespoon brown sugar
4 tablespoons peanut or canola oil
24 ounces (720 g) uncooked boneless skinless chicken breasts, cut into thin strips
2 carrots, peeled and julienned
2 red bell peppers, julienned
2 cups small broccoli florets
4 cloves garlic, minced
4 teaspoons finely grated fresh ginger
2 cups chicken or vegetable stock
2 tablespoons cornstarch (corn flour), mixed to a paste with 2 tablespoons water

Add the dried noodles to a saucepan of boiling water and cook for 5 minutes. While the noodles cook, mix together the soy sauce, oyster sauce, Chinese rice wine, sesame oil, five-spice powder, and sugar in a small bowl.

Heat a wok or large skillet over high heat, add 2 tablespoons of the peanut oil, and stir-fry the chicken for 4 minutes. Remove the chicken from the wok and set aside on a plate. Heat the remaining oil in the wok, and stir-fry the carrots, bell peppers, and broccoli for 4 minutes. Add the garlic and ginger and stir-fry for 1 minute, then return the chicken to the wok. Add the sauce mixture and stock and cook for 1 minute. Add the cornstarch paste and cook until thickened and thoroughly combined. Serve on a bed of the noodles.

VARIATION: Use shrimp, scallops, or cubed firm tofu in place of the chicken. Rice can be served instead of noodles.

Shrimp, Bok Choy, and Snow Pea Stir-Fry

We've found that bok choy combines perfectly with snow peas and shrimp. So, not surprisingly, this is one of our favorite stir-fry dishes.

SERVES 4

2 cups long-grain white rice

6 tablespoons oyster sauce

4 tablespoons soy sauce

2 tablespoons Chinese rice wine (or dry sherry)

2 tablespoons water

2 teaspoons sesame oil

1 tablespoon brown sugar

4 tablespoons peanut or canola oil

32 large uncooked shrimp (prawns), peeled

2 red bell peppers, julienned

2 bunches bok choy, roughly chopped

32 snow peas, trimmed and halved on the diagonal

4 cloves garlic, minced

Bring 3 cups of water to a boil in a saucepan. Stir in the rice, and keep stirring until the water returns to a boil. Cover the pot with a tight-fitting lid, reduce the heat to very low, and simmer gently for 15 minutes.

While the rice cooks, mix together the oyster sauce, soy sauce, Chinese rice wine, water, sesame oil, and sugar in a small bowl.

Heat a wok or large skillet over high heat, add 2 tablespoons of the peanut oil, and stir-fry the shrimp for 2 minutes. Remove the shrimp from the wok and set aside on a plate. Heat the remaining oil in the wok and stir-fry the bell pepper for 2 minutes. Add the bok choy and snow peas and stir-fry for 4 minutes. Add the garlic and stir-fry for 1 minute, then return the shrimp to the wok. Add the sauce mixture and mix to heat through. Serve with the rice.

Thai Chicken Stir-Fry

Strips of chicken and a selection of tasty vegetables are stir-fried with Thai seasonings and accented with crunchy crushed peanuts.

SERVES 4

2 cups jasmine white rice

6 tablespoons fish sauce

4 tablespoons freshly squeezed lemon juice

2 teaspoons brown sugar

4 teaspoons sesame oil

5 tablespoons peanut or canola oil

24 ounces (720 g) boneless skinless chicken breasts, cut into thin strips

2 green bell peppers, julienned

4 cloves garlic, finely chopped

4 teaspoons Thai red curry paste

4 ripe tomatoes, diced

1 cup frozen peas, thawed

4 scallions (white and green parts), trimmed and thinly sliced on the diagonal; reserve a little for garnish

A handful of cilantro (fresh coriander) leaves; reserve a little for garnish

4 tablespoons crushed roasted peanuts

Bring 3 cups of water to a boil in a saucepan. Stir in the rice, and keep stirring until the water returns to a boil. Cover the pot with a tight-fitting lid, reduce the heat to very low, and simmer gently for 15 minutes.

While the rice cooks, mix together the fish sauce, lemon juice, sugar, and sesame oil in a small bowl. Heat a wok or large skillet over high heat, add 2 tablespoons of the peanut oil, and stir-fry the chicken for 3 minutes; remove from the wok and set aside on a plate. Add the remaining oil to the hot wok and stir-fry the bell pepper for 3 minutes. Add the garlic and curry paste and stir-fry for 30 seconds, until the curry paste has dissolved. Add the tomatoes and peas and stir-fry for 1 minute. Add the sauce mixture, scallions, and chicken and heat through. Stir through the cilantro and peanuts, and serve over rice garnished with the reserved scallions and cilantro.

Honey-Lemon Chicken with Almonds

In this tasty Chinese dish, a mixture of soy sauce, hoisin sauce, lemon juice, and honey coats succulent chicken pieces and vegetables with a sweet and savory glaze.

SERVES 4

8 ounces (240 g) dried wheat noodles
6 tablespoons freshly squeezed lemon juice
6 tablespoons soy sauce
3 tablespoons honey
2 tablespoons hoisin sauce
4 tablespoons canola or peanut oil
24 ounces (720 g) uncooked boneless skinless chicken breasts, cut into strips
4 cups broccoli florets
2 red bell peppers, julienned
1 stick celery, finely sliced on the diagonal
4 tablespoons sliced almonds
4 cloves garlic, minced
4 teaspoons finely grated fresh ginger
3 cups chicken stock
3 tablespoons cornstarch (corn flour), mixed to a paste with 3 tablespoons water

Bring a saucepan of water to a boil. Add the dried noodles to the boiling water and cook for 5 minutes.

While the noodles cook, mix together the lemon juice, soy sauce, honey, and hoisin sauce in a bowl. Heat a wok or large skillet over high heat, add 2 tablespoons of the oil, and stir-fry the chicken for 3 minutes. Remove the chicken from the wok and set aside on a plate. Heat the remaining oil in the wok and stir-fry the broccoli, bell pepper, and celery for 6 minutes. Add the sliced almonds and stir-fry for another minute. Add the garlic and ginger and stir-fry for 1 minute, then return the chicken to the wok. Add the sauce mixture and stock, then add the cornstarch paste and cook, stirring continuously, until thickened. Serve on a bed of the noodles.

VARIATION: Replace the chicken with shrimp, scallops, or fish.

Stir-Fried Beef in Black Bean Sauce

Tender beef strips and vegetables in a rich black bean sauce. Stir-frying is a great way to make a little red meat stretch a long way.

SERVES 4

2 cups long-grain white rice

6 tablespoons black bean sauce

4 tablespoons soy sauce

2 tablespoons Chinese rice wine

4 teaspoons brown sugar

1 teaspoon ground black pepper

4 tablespoons canola or peanut oil

24 ounces (720 g) lean beef, cut into thin strips along the grain

24 green beans, ends trimmed, cut in ½ on the diagonal

2 red bell peppers, julienned

2 onions, each cut into 8 wedges and separated into pieces

6 cloves garlic, minced

4 teaspoons finely grated fresh ginger

3 cups beef stock

3 tablespoons cornstarch (corn flour), mixed to a paste with 3 tablespoons water

Bring 3 cups of water to a boil in a saucepan. Stir in the rice, and keep stirring until the water returns to a boil. Cover the pot with a tight-fitting lid, reduce the heat to very low, and simmer gently for 15 minutes.

While the rice cooks, mix together the black bean sauce, soy sauce, Chinese rice wine, sugar, and black pepper in a bowl. Heat a wok or large skillet over high heat, add 2 tablespoons of the oil, and stir-fry the beef for 5 minutes. Remove the beef from the wok and set aside on a plate. Heat the remaining oil in the wok and stir-fry the green beans, bell peppers, and onions for 7 minutes. Add the garlic and ginger and stir-fry for another minute, then return the beef to the wok. Add the sauce mixture and stock, then add the cornstarch paste and cook, stirring continuously, until thickened. Serve on a bed of the rice.

VARIATION: This black bean sauce also goes well with chicken, lean pork, squid, shrimp, or bite-sized pieces of firm whitefish.

Indonesian Stir-Fried Tempeh and Vegetables

Made from fermented soybeans, tempeh has a nutty flavor and a firm, meaty texture. Here it's combined with red pepper and snow peas to make a simple and satisfying Indonesian-style stir-fry.

SERVES 4

2 cups long-grain white rice

4 tablespoons *kecap manis* (Indonesian sweet soy sauce)

4 tablespoons soy sauce

4 tablespoons water

2 teaspoons tamarind puree

4 tablespoons canola or peanut oil

14 ounces (420 g) tempeh, cut into small cubes

2 red bell peppers, julienned

32 snow peas, ends trimmed

4 cloves garlic, finely chopped

2 tablespoons finely grated fresh ginger

2 scallions (white and green parts), trimmed and thinly sliced on the diagonal

4 tablespoons roughly torn cilantro (fresh coriander) leaves

Bring 3 cups of water to a boil in a saucepan. Stir in the rice, and keep stirring until the water returns to a boil. Cover the pot with a tight-fitting lid, reduce the heat to very low, and simmer gently for 15 minutes.

While the rice cooks, mix together the *kecap manis*, soy sauce, water, and tamarind puree in a small bowl. Heat the oil in a wok or large skillet over high heat, add the tempeh, bell pepper, and snow peas and stir-fry for 5 minutes. Add the garlic and ginger and stir-fry for 1 minute. Add the sauce mix, scallions, and cilantro and stir-fry for 30 seconds. Serve with the rice.

Ginger-Steamed Fish with Stir-Fried Vegetables

Fish is steamed over ginger-infused water and served with stir-fried vegetables and noodles.

4 tablespoons soy sauce

2 tablespoons oyster sauce

2 tablespoons hoisin sauce

2 tablespoons Chinese rice wine

2-inch piece of fresh ginger, peeled

Four 6-ounce (180 g) uncooked firm whitefish fillets
  (such as snapper, cod, or haddock)

8 ounces (240 g) dried wheat noodles

2 tablespoons peanut or canola oil

2 carrots, peeled and julienned

2 zucchini (courgettes), julienned

4 scallions (white and green parts), trimmed and thinly sliced on the diagonal

4 cloves garlic, minced

4 teaspoons finely grated fresh ginger

3 cups chicken stock

3 tablespoons cornstarch (corn flour), mixed to a paste with 3 tablespoons water

Bring a saucepan of water to a boil.

Mix together the soy sauce, oyster sauce, hoisin sauce, and Chinese rice wine in a bowl. Crush the ginger with the side of a large knife blade. Place the crushed ginger in the water in the bottom of a steamer pan and bring to a boil. Place the fish in a lightly oiled steamer basket, place over the boiling water, cover with the lid, and steam for 10 minutes.

While the fish steams, cook the noodles in the saucepan of boiling water for 5 minutes.

While the noodles cook, heat a wok or large skillet over high heat, add the oil, and stir-fry the carrots for 3 minutes. Add the zucchini and stir-fry for 3 minutes. Add the scallion, garlic, and ginger and stir-fry for another minute. Add the sauce mixture and stock, then add the cornstarch paste and cook, stirring continuously, until thickened. Add the drained cooked noodles and thoroughly combine. Break the steamed fish into pieces and gently fold into the vegetables and noodles.

TIP: If you don't have a steamer pan, heat the water in the bottom of a wok over high heat until boiling and place the fish on a plate, then on a steamer rack or upturned cup in the wok. Cover with the lid and steam as directed.

Five-Spice Squid

This dish combines quick-cooking squid and vegetables with a rich sauce laced with fragrant Chinese five-spice powder. Scoring the squid makes the pieces curl up when cooked.

SERVES 4

2 cups long-grain white rice
4 tablespoons hoisin sauce
4 tablespoons soy sauce
2 tablespoons Chinese rice wine
2 teaspoons brown sugar
1 teaspoon five-spice powder
2 teaspoons sesame oil
6 tablespoons canola or peanut oil
4 cleaned squid hoods, each cut in half, scored on the inside in a crisscross pattern,
     and cut into large pieces
2 red bell peppers, julienned
2 bunches Asian greens (such as bok choy or choy sum), roughly chopped
4 cloves garlic, minced
2 teaspoons finely grated fresh ginger
2 small red chiles, deseeded and finely chopped
3 cups fish, chicken, or vegetable stock
3 tablespoons cornstarch (corn flour), mixed to a paste with 3 tablespoons water

Bring 3 cups of water to a boil in a saucepan. Stir in the rice, and keep stirring until the water returns to a boil. Cover the pot with a tight-fitting lid, reduce the heat to very low, and simmer gently for 15 minutes.

While the rice cooks, mix together the hoisin sauce, soy sauce, Chinese rice wine, sugar, five-spice powder, and sesame oil in a bowl.

Heat a wok or large skillet over high heat, add 2 tablespoons of the peanut oil, and stir-fry the squid for 40 seconds. Remove the squid from the wok and set aside on a plate. Heat the remaining oil in the wok over high heat and stir-fry the bell peppers for 2 minutes. Add the Asian greens and stir-fry for another 3 minutes. Add the garlic, ginger, and chiles and stir-fry for 1 minute. Add the sauce mixture and stock, then add the cornstarch paste and cook, stirring continuously, until thickened. Return the squid to the wok and thoroughly combine. Serve with the rice.

Pizza

Traditional Italian pizza is markedly different from a typical Western pizza. For a start, a thick doughy crust isn't traditional. Instead, a thin crust—which contains far fewer calories—is the usual choice. Meaty toppings certainly aren't traditional either. Instead, popular toppings include fresh herbs (like torn basil), anchovies, olives, bell peppers, and mushrooms. And traditional pizza isn't smothered in cheese; only a moderate amount is used, simply to accent the flavors of the toppings. So pizza made the Italian way ends up containing far fewer calories and bad fats than typical Western pizza, which means you can enjoy it without guilt (especially if you enjoy it with a fresh salad on the side). Below is a "master recipe" for pizza, followed by a number of variations.

▶ Basic Pizza recipe

SERVES 2

3 tablespoons chopped canned whole tomatoes
1 tablespoon tomato paste
½ clove garlic, minced
1 teaspoon extra-virgin olive oil
½ teaspoon salt
¼ teaspoon freshly ground black pepper
1 store-bought prebaked pizza crust (about 12 inches in diameter and
    preferably thin crust, or a large whole-grain pita bread)
Toppings (topping variations follow)
2½ ounces (75 g) mozzarella cheese, cut into small cubes or grated

Preheat the oven to 450°F (230°C).

In a small bowl, mix together the tomatoes, tomato paste, garlic, olive oil, salt and pepper. Spread a thin layer evenly over the pizza crust. Arrange the toppings evenly over the pizza crust. Place the cubed cheese evenly on top. Place the pizza on a pizza pan and cook for 10 minutes. Cut into 6 slices to serve.

Pizza Toppings

ANCHOVY, OLIVE, AND BASIL PIZZA

4 large fresh basil leaves, roughly torn

5 anchovy fillets, chopped

8 pitted black olives, halved

SMOKED SALMON PIZZA

3½ ounces (100 g) sliced smoked salmon, cut into strips

12 capers, rinsed and drained

¼ green bell pepper, diced

6 thinly sliced red onion rings

BROCCOLI, TUNA, BLUE CHEESE, AND WALNUT PIZZA

6 ounces (180 g) canned tuna in olive oil, drained and broken into chunks

⅓ cup lightly crushed walnuts

1½ cups small broccoli florets, steamed over simmering water for 3 minutes

1½ ounces (45 g) crumbled blue cheese, such as Gorgonzola

SICILIAN TUNA AND BASIL PIZZA

5 large fresh basil leaves, roughly torn

½ green bell pepper, finely sliced

6 ounces (180 g) canned light tuna in olive oil, drained and broken into small chunks

EARTH AND SEA PIZZA

8 peeled uncooked large shrimp (prawns)

8 large scallops

6 thinly sliced red onion rings

½ red bell pepper, finely diced

5 black olives, sliced

HAM, MUSHROOM, AND TOMATO PIZZA

2 ripe tomatoes, thinly sliced

2 white button mushrooms, sliced

2 thin slices ham, diced

continues on next page

PESTO CHICKEN PIZZA

3 tablespoons Pesto Genoese (page 278) or store-bought pesto spread
   over the crust instead of the tomato sauce mix
2 ripe tomatoes, thinly sliced
1 cup shredded, precooked skinless chicken breast
6 thinly sliced red onion rings
8 pitted black olives, thinly sliced

GREEK PIZZA WITH CHICKEN, ARTICHOKES, AND FETA

1 cup shredded, precooked skinless chicken breast
1 handful fresh spinach leaves, roughly chopped
2 jarred marinated artichoke hearts, quartered
1/4 red bell pepper, diced
6 pitted kalamata olives, thinly sliced
2 1/2 ounces (75 g) feta cheese, crumbled (used in place of the mozzarella cheese)

THAI SHRIMP PIZZA

4 tablespoons sweet chili sauce spread over the crust instead of the tomato sauce mix
12 peeled uncooked large shrimp (prawns)
1/4 red bell pepper, diced
1/4 green bell pepper, diced
1 scallion (white and green parts), trimmed and thinly sliced

ANCHOVY, OLIVE, AND
BASIL PIZZA (PAGE 169)

CHAKCHOUKA (PAGE 264)

EARTH AND SEA PIZZA
(PAGE 169)

JAPANESE-STYLE
MARINATED GRILLED
TUNA (PAGE 216),
JAPANESE SOBA
NOODLE SALAD
(PAGE 252)

SAVORY SALMON SPREAD
(PAGE 290)

MEDITERRANEAN-STYLE GRILLED
MARINATED SALMON (PAGE 218)

SHRIMP, TOMATO,
PEA, AND BASIL
RISOTTO
(PAGE 186)

MUSHROOM BRUSCHETTA
(PAGE 236)

SALMON KEDGEREE
(PAGE 190)

PAN BAGNAT (PAGE 238)

PANZANELLA (PAGE 258)

FOCACCIA WITH
SMOKED SALMON AND
AVOCADO (PAGE 232)

PASTA PRIMAVERA
(PAGE 145)

PASTA
PUTTANESCA
(PAGE 144)

PASTA WITH
TUNA, GREEN
BEANS, OLIVES,
AND ROMESCO
SAUCE
(PAGE 154)

TOFU AND CASHEW CHOW MEIN (PAGE 198)

STIR-FRIED BEEF IN BLACK BEAN SAUCE (PAGE 162

HUMMUS (PAGE 284)

PESTO GENOESE (PAGE 278), ROMESCO SAUCE
(PAGE 283), AND BABA GHANOUSH (PAGE 286)

THAI-SPICED SWEET POTATO SOUP (PAGE 249)

TERIYAKI CHICKEN NOODLES (PAGE 199)   SHRIMP FRIED RICE (PAGE 193)

THAI FISH CAKES WITH SWEET CHILI SAUCE (PAGE 274)

NUOC CHAM DIPPING SAUCE (PAGE 284), INDONESIAN PEANUT SAUCE (PAGE 282), CHINESE-STYLE DIPPING SAUCE (PAGE 288), AND SESAME-HOISIN DIPPING SAUCE (PAGE 288)

GREEK FAVA BEAN, EGGPLANT, AND OLIVE STEW WITH FETA (PAGE 182)

SUSHI ROLLS (PAGE 206)

ASIAN-STYLE FRUIT SALAD (PAGE 296)

MIXED BERRY COULIS WITH GREEK
VANILLA YOGURT (PAGE 292)

PROVENÇAL APPLE AND WALNUT PIE
(PAGE 294)

TUNISIAN ORANGE, DATE, AND
PISTACHIO SALAD (PAGE 295)

GREEK SALAD (PAGE 253)

GADO GADO (PAGE 259)

INSALATA DI RISO (PAGE 255)

TABBOULEH (PAGE 257)   SALADE NIÇOISE (PAGE 254)

FAVA BEANS WITH MARINATED ARTICHOKE HEARTS AND OLIVES (PAGE 273)

MALAYSIAN FISH LAKSA
(PAGE 200)

SHRIMP, BOK CHOY, AND SNOW
PEA STIR-FRY (PAGE 159)

VIETNAMESE BAKED FISH
(PAGE 183)

TUNISIAN
CHICKEN
AND
ALMOND
COUSCOUS
(PAGE 192)

MUSHROOM, BACON, AND
WALNUT RISOTTO (PAGE 189)

THAI RED CHICKEN
CURRY (PAGE 172)

FRESH TUNA
AND VEGETABLE
SKEWERS
(PAGE 219)

CREAMY CHICKEN,
MUSHROOM, AND SUN-
DRIED TOMATO PASTA
(PAGE 153)

MINESTRONE
SOUP
(PAGE 240)

FIVE-SPICE SQUID (PAGE 166)

GREEK SPINACH AND WHITE
BEAN SOUP (PAGE 246)

SOUTH
INDIAN
SHRIMP
CURRY
(PAGE 174)

CHICKEN CACCIATORE (PAGE 178)

THAI CHICKEN STIR-FRY (PAGE 160)

Curries,
Stews, and
Baked Dishes

Thai Red Chicken Curry

A traditional Thai curry made with a subtle blend of hot, salty, sweet, and sour flavors to get the taste buds tingling. You can make your own curry paste from scratch, but to save time we recommend you buy a good-quality premade Thai curry paste.

SERVES 4

4 tablespoons canola or peanut oil

2 onions, finely chopped

4 teaspoons Thai red curry paste (or 6 teaspoons for a hotter curry)

4 cloves garlic, finely chopped

2 cups coconut milk

2 cups chicken stock

4 tablespoons fish sauce

2 tablespoons brown sugar

1 teaspoon salt

2 zucchini (courgettes), sliced into thin rounds

2 red bell peppers, julienned

2 cups jasmine white rice

24 ounces (720 g) uncooked skinless chicken breast fillets, cut into bite-size pieces

4 tablespoons cornstarch (corn flour), mixed to a paste with 4 tablespoons water

4 tablespoons freshly squeezed lemon juice

8 large fresh basil leaves, finely sliced

Heat the oil in a large saucepan over medium heat and cook the onions, stirring occasionally, until softened, about 5 minutes. Add the curry paste and garlic and cook, stirring, for 1 minute. Add the coconut milk, stock, fish sauce, sugar, and salt, then bring to a boil. Add the zucchini and bell peppers, cover with a lid, reduce the heat to medium, and simmer for 12 minutes.

While the curry simmers, bring 3 cups of water to a boil in a saucepan. Stir in the rice, and keep stirring until the water returns to a boil. Cover the pot with a tight-fitting lid, reduce the heat to very low, and simmer gently for 15 minutes.

Add the chicken to the curry and simmer, covered, for another 8 minutes. Add the cornstarch paste and stir continuously until the curry thickens, then stir in the lemon juice and basil. Serve on a bed of the rice.

VARIATIONS: This curry tastes equally delicious using any selection of seafood, such as shrimp, scallops, or pieces of firm fish or cubed firm tofu.

You can also use a variety of different vegetables with this curry, including shredded cabbage, thinly sliced carrots, or green beans. Be flexible and adapt the recipe to make the most of seasonal produce.

South Indian Shrimp Curry

Some of the greatest seafood curries originate along the south coast of India where shrimp, fish, and other seafood are plentiful. In this shrimp curry, a fragrant spice mix imparts a deep color and encapsulates the rich flavors of South Indian cuisine.

SERVES 4

4 tablespoons canola or peanut oil
2 onions, chopped
4 cloves garlic, finely chopped
2 teaspoons finely grated fresh ginger
4 teaspoons ground cumin
3 teaspoons turmeric
2 teaspoons paprika
1 teaspoon chili powder
2 cups canned whole tomatoes, chopped
2 cups coconut milk
2 teaspoons salt
2 cups basmati rice
32 large uncooked shrimp (prawns), peeled and deveined
4 tablespoons chopped cilantro (fresh coriander)
4 tablespoons freshly squeezed lemon juice

Heat the oil in a large saucepan over medium heat and cook the onions, stirring occasionally, until golden, about 8 minutes. Add the garlic, ginger, cumin, turmeric, paprika, and chili powder and cook, stirring, for 1 minute. Add the tomatoes, coconut milk, and salt and bring to a boil. Reduce the heat to medium and simmer, uncovered, for 8 minutes.

While the curry simmers, bring 3 cups of water to a boil in a saucepan. Stir in the rice and keep stirring until the water returns to a boil. Cover the pot with a tight-fitting lid, reduce the heat to very low, and simmer gently for 15 minutes.

Add the shrimp and cilantro to the curry, cover with a lid, simmer for another 4 minutes, then stir in the lemon juice. Serve on a bed of the rice.

SERVING IDEA: This curry tastes particularly good served with the classic Indian accompaniment Raita (page 280).

TIP: You can substitute large precooked, peeled shrimp for the fresh shrimp. Add them during the last minute of cooking to heat through.

Dahl with Carrot and Cauliflower

A traditional Indian dahl (lentil curry) with carrots and cauliflower, served on a bed of basmati rice. Lentils are a good source of protein and fiber, and they cook quickly into a thick and creamy puree. Dahl is usually eaten with rice or Indian breads, like naan or chapati, to soak up the delicious and nutritious gravy.

SERVES 4

3 tablespoons peanut or canola oil
2 onions, chopped
2 carrots, quartered lengthways and thinly sliced
4 cloves garlic, finely chopped
1 tablespoon finely grated fresh ginger
$1\frac{1}{2}$ teaspoons ground coriander
$1\frac{1}{2}$ teaspoons ground cumin
1 teaspoon turmeric
$\frac{3}{4}$ teaspoon cinnamon
$\frac{3}{4}$ teaspoon chili powder
2 cups cauliflower florets
$1\frac{1}{2}$ cups red lentils
14 ounces (420 g) canned tomatoes, chopped
$1\frac{1}{2}$ cups coconut milk
$1\frac{1}{2}$ cups vegetable or chicken stock
$1\frac{1}{2}$ teaspoons salt
2 cups basmati rice
2 tablespoons freshly squeezed lemon juice

Heat the oil in a large saucepan over medium heat and cook the onions and carrots, stirring occasionally, until softened, about 8 minutes. Add the garlic, ginger, coriander, cumin, turmeric, cinnamon, and chili powder and cook, stirring, for 1 minute. Add the cauliflower and red lentils and stir to coat them with the spice mixture. Add the tomatoes, coconut milk, stock, and salt, bring to a boil, and cover with a lid. Reduce the heat to medium and simmer for 20 minutes, stirring occasionally.

While the dahl simmers, bring 3 cups of water to a boil in a saucepan. Stir in the rice, and keep stirring until the water returns to a boil. Cover the pot with a tight-fitting lid, reduce the heat to very low, and simmer gently for 15 minutes.

Remove the dahl from the heat and stir in the lemon juice. Serve on a bed of the basmati rice.

Fragrant Chicken Curry

With a few key ingredients stocked in your pantry (such as spices, canned tomatoes, and coconut milk) and a selection of vegetables, it's easy to produce authentic Indian curries in your own kitchen. Like most curries, this recipe is simple, doesn't involve a lot of steps, and simmers away with no effort required, filling the kitchen with mouthwatering aromas.

SERVES 4

4 tablespoons canola oil
2 onions, chopped
4 cloves garlic, finely chopped
2 teaspoons finely grated fresh ginger
2 teaspoons turmeric
2 teaspoons ground cumin
1 teaspoon chili powder
2 cups canned whole tomatoes, chopped
2 cups coconut milk
3 teaspoons garam masala
2 teaspoons salt
2 cups basmati rice
24 ounces (720 g) uncooked skinless chicken breast fillets, cut into bite-size pieces
1 cup frozen green peas, thawed
2 tablespoons freshly squeezed lemon juice
2 tablespoons finely chopped fresh cilantro (fresh coriander)

Heat the oil in a frying pan over medium heat and cook the onions, stirring occasionally, until golden, about 8 minutes. Add the garlic and cook, stirring, for 2 minutes. Add the ginger, turmeric, cumin, and chili powder and cook, stirring, for 1 minute. Add the tomatoes, coconut milk, garam masala, and salt and bring to a boil. Reduce the heat to medium and simmer for 8 minutes.

While the curry simmers, bring 3 cups of water to a boil in a saucepan. Stir in the rice and keep stirring until the water returns to a boil. Cover the pot with a tight-fitting lid, reduce the heat to very low, and simmer gently for 15 minutes.

Add the chicken and peas to the curry, cover with a lid, and simmer for another 8 minutes, then stir in the lemon juice and cilantro. Serve on a bed of the rice.

VARIATION: Replace the chicken with seafood such as shrimp or scallops.

Thai Fish Curry

A fragrant, richly flavored fish curry with green beans and red pepper and served with jasmine rice.

SERVES 4

4 tablespoons canola or peanut oil
1 red bell pepper, julienned
32 green beans, trimmed and halved
4 cloves garlic, finely chopped
2 teaspoons finely chopped lemongrass
2 teaspoons finely grated fresh ginger
2 teaspoons turmeric
2 cups coconut milk
1 cup water
4 tablespoons fish sauce
4 teaspoons brown sugar
1 teaspoon chili powder
2 cups jasmine white rice
Four 6-ounce (180 g) firm whitefish fillets (such as snapper, cod, or haddock), each cut into thirds
2 tablespoons freshly squeezed lemon juice
2 tablespoons finely chopped fresh basil

Heat the oil in a large skillet over medium heat, and cook the bell pepper and green beans, stirring occasionally, until the pepper is softened, about 4 minutes. Add the garlic, lemongrass, ginger, and turmeric and cook, stirring constantly, for 1 minute. Add the coconut milk, water, fish sauce, sugar, and chili powder and bring to a boil. Reduce the heat to medium and simmer for 8 minutes.

While the curry simmers, bring 3 cups of water to a boil in a saucepan. Stir in the rice and keep stirring until the water returns to a boil. Cover the pot with a tight-fitting lid, reduce the heat to very low, and simmer gently for 15 minutes.

Add the fish, spooning the curry sauce over the fish to coat, and simmer, covered, for 8 minutes. Remove from the heat and stir in the lemon juice and basil. Serve with the rice.

Chicken Cacciatore

In this classic Italian dish, tender chicken breast fillets are coated with a flavorful sauce made with tomatoes, anchovies, olives, and wine and seasoned with oregano and balsamic vinegar.

SERVES 4

2 cups long-grain white rice
6 tablespoons extra-virgin olive oil
Four 6-ounce (180 g) uncooked skinless chicken breast fillets
2 onions, chopped
1 red bell pepper, julienned
4 cloves garlic, finely chopped
4 anchovy fillets, finely chopped
14-ounce (420 g) canned whole tomatoes, chopped
1 cup white wine
2 tablespoons tomato paste
2 tablespoons balsamic vinegar
16 black pitted olives, quartered
1 teaspoon dried oregano
1 teaspoon sea salt
½ teaspoon freshly ground black pepper
4 teaspoons finely chopped fresh flat-leaf parsley

Bring 3 cups of water to a boil in a saucepan. Stir in the rice, and keep stirring until the water returns to a boil. Cover the pot with a tight-fitting lid, reduce the heat to very low, and simmer gently for 15 minutes.

While the rice is cooking, heat 2 tablespoons of the olive oil in a large skillet over medium-high heat. Cook the chicken for 3 minutes on each side, then remove from pan and set aside on a plate. Heat the reserved oil in the same pan, and cook the onions and bell pepper, stirring occasionally, until softened, about 5 minutes. Add the garlic and anchovies and cook 1 minute more, stirring to break up the anchovies. Add the tomatoes, white wine, tomato paste, vinegar, olives, oregano, salt, and pepper and simmer over medium heat, covered, for 10 minutes. Return the chicken fillets to the pan and cook for 3 minutes. Serve on a bed of the rice, garnished with the parsley.

Greek Shrimp with Feta

This appetizing and richly flavored dish echoes the traditional flavors of Greek cuisine.

SERVES 4

6 tablespoons extra-virgin olive oil
2 onions, finely chopped
2 green bell peppers, diced
4 scallions (white and green parts), trimmed and thinly sliced
6 cloves garlic, finely chopped
28 ounces (840 g) canned whole tomatoes, chopped
1 cup white wine
1 teaspoon dried oregano
2 teaspoons sea salt
1 teaspoon freshly ground black pepper
2 cups long-grain white rice
24 large uncooked shrimp, peeled and deveined
4 tablespoons chopped fresh flat-leaf parsley
5 ounces (150 g) crumbled feta cheese

Heat 4 tablespoons of the oil in an ovenproof skillet over medium heat, and cook the onions and bell peppers, stirring occasionally, until softened, about 5 minutes. Add the scallions and garlic and cook, stirring, for another 2 minutes. Add the tomatoes, wine, oregano, salt, and pepper and bring to a boil. Reduce the heat to medium and simmer for 10 minutes.

Bring 3 cups of water to a boil in a saucepan. Stir in the rice, and keep stirring until the water returns to a boil. Cover the pot with a tight-fitting lid, reduce the heat to very low, and simmer gently for 15 minutes.

Add the shrimp, parsley, and reserved oil to the stew and simmer, covered, for another 3 minutes. Sprinkle the feta cheese on top and place the skillet under a hot oven broiler to brown the feta, about 2 minutes. Serve with the rice.

Spanish Tuna and Vegetable Stew

Spanish cuisine makes the most of foods from the land and the sea, and this traditional recipe combines the best of both.

SERVES 4

6 tablespoons extra-virgin olive oil
2 red onions, finely chopped
1 red bell pepper, julienned
1 green bell pepper, julienned
28 ounces (840 g) canned whole tomatoes, chopped
2 small potatoes, peeled and cut into small cubes
6 cloves garlic, finely chopped
3 cups fish, vegetable, or chicken stock
1 cup white wine
2 tablespoons tomato paste
4 teaspoons paprika
2 teaspoon sea salt
1 teaspoon freshly ground black pepper
2 cups long-grain white rice
12 ounces (360 g) canned light tuna, drained and broken into small chunks
2 tablespoons finely chopped fresh flat-leaf parsley

Heat 4 tablespoons of the oil in a large saucepan over medium heat, and cook the onions and bell peppers, stirring occasionally, until softened, about 6 minutes. Add the tomatoes, potatoes, and garlic and cook, stirring, for 2 minutes. Add the stock, wine, tomato paste, paprika, salt, and pepper and bring to a boil. Reduce the heat to medium high and simmer, stirring occasionally, for 25 minutes.

While the stew simmers, bring 3 cups of water to a boil in a saucepan. Stir in the rice, and keep stirring until the water returns to a boil. Cover the pot with a tight-fitting lid, reduce the heat to very low, and simmer gently for 15 minutes.

Stir the tuna, parsley, and reserved oil into the stew and serve over the rice.

VARIATION: Instead of rice, you can serve this stew with good-quality crusty bread.

Moroccan Stew with Couscous

An abundance of nourishing ingredients including chickpeas, cabbage, sweet potatoes, and green beans are simmered in a delicately spiced tomato-peanut sauce and served with fluffy couscous.

SERVES 4

3 tablespoons extra-virgin olive oil
2 onions, finely chopped
3 cloves garlic, finely chopped
2 teaspoons finely grated fresh ginger
½ teaspoon chili powder
1½ cups of green beans, ends trimmed and cut in half
2 sweet potatoes, peeled and cut into bite-size cubes
3 cups shredded cabbage
2 cups canned whole tomatoes, chopped
4 tablespoons natural peanut butter
2 cups vegetable or chicken stock
2 teaspoons salt
1½ cups canned chickpeas, rinsed and drained
2 cups couscous
3 tablespoons freshly squeezed lemon juice
3 tablespoons chopped cilantro (fresh coriander)

Heat the oil in a large saucepan over medium heat, and cook the onions, stirring occasionally, until softened, about 5 minutes. Add the garlic, ginger, and chili powder and cook, stirring, for 1 minute. Add the green beans, sweet potatoes, cabbage, tomatoes, peanut butter, stock, and 1 teaspoon salt and bring to a boil. Reduce the heat to medium and simmer for 15 minutes. Add the chickpeas and simmer for 10 minutes.

While the stew simmers, mix 2½ cups of boiling water and 1 teaspoon of salt with the couscous in a bowl. Cover with a dish towel or plate to seal in the steam and let sit for 5 minutes. Fluff with a fork to separate the grains.

Stir the lemon juice and cilantro into the stew and serve with the couscous.

VARIATIONS: Garnish with sliced boiled eggs; replace the sweet potato with pumpkin; use spinach instead of cabbage.

Greek Fava Bean, Eggplant, and Olive Stew with Feta

A richly flavored Greek stew with fava beans, eggplant, zucchini, red pepper, potatoes, and kalamata olives, served with crumbled feta cheese.

SERVES 4

5 tablespoons extra-virgin olive oil

2 red onions, diced

1 eggplant (aubergine), cut into small cubes

1 red bell pepper, diced

1 zucchini (courgette), diced

1 potato, cut into small cubes

6 cloves garlic, minced

1 teaspoon dried oregano

28 ounces (840 g) canned whole tomatoes, chopped

2 cups chicken or vegetable stock

2 teaspoons salt

1 teaspoon freshly ground black pepper

2 cups bulgur

8 ounces (240 g) frozen fava (broad) beans, cooked in boiling water for 5 minutes, rinsed under cold water, skins removed.

4 tablespoons finely chopped fresh flat-leaf parsley

24 pitted kalamata olives, halved

4 ounces (120 g) feta cheese

Heat 3 tablespoons of the oil in a large saucepan and cook the onions, stirring occasionally, until lightly browned, about 8 minutes. Add the eggplant, bell pepper, and zucchini and cook, stirring, for 5 minutes. Add the potato, garlic, and oregano and cook, stirring, for 1 minute. Add the tomatoes, stock, salt, and pepper; stir well to combine and bring to a boil. Reduce the heat to medium and cook, stirring occasionally, for 20 minutes.

While the stew simmers, mix the bulgur with 3 cups of water in a saucepan. Bring to a boil, cover, then turn the heat on very low and cook for 15 minutes. Fluff with a fork to separate the grains. Add the cooked, peeled fava beans, parsley, and olives to the stew and cook for 10 minutes. Remove from the heat and stir in the reserved 2 tablespoons of olive oil. Serve over the bulgur with crumbled feta cheese on top.

Vietnamese Baked Fish

Tender fillets of fish combined with chopped tomatoes, fresh mint, and Vietnamese-style seasonings, then baked in foil to infuse the flavors.

SERVES 4

4 ripe tomatoes, diced
4 tablespoons fish sauce
2 tablespoons freshly squeezed lemon juice
2 teaspoons sesame oil
4 teaspoons finely grated fresh ginger
2 cloves garlic, finely chopped
2 tablespoons finely chopped fresh mint
1 teaspoon sugar
½ teaspoon black pepper
Four 6-ounce (180 g) fillets firm whitefish (such as snapper, cod, or haddock)
2 carrots, julienned
2 cups long-grain white rice

Preheat the oven to 440°F (225°C).

In a bowl, mix together the tomatoes, fish sauce, lemon juice, sesame oil, ginger, garlic, mint, sugar, and pepper until well combined. Place a fish fillet in the center of each of four 12-inch pieces of foil and arrange the carrots on top. Spoon equal amounts of the tomato mixture over each. Fold the foil over the fish and vegetables and seal the foil packets tightly (fold the edges together so no steam can escape). Place the packets on a baking sheet and bake in the oven for 16 minutes.

While the fish cooks, bring 3 cups of water to a boil in a saucepan. Stir in the rice, and keep stirring until the water returns to a boil. Cover the pot with a tight-fitting lid, reduce the heat to very low, and simmer gently for 15 minutes.

Remove the packets from the oven and open (be careful—the steam is very hot). Transfer the fish, vegetables, and sauce from the foil packets to serving plates and accompany with the rice.

TIP: These foil packets can be prepared in advance and left to marinate in the fridge until you're ready to cook.

Provençal Baked Fish with Vegetables

Provence is a region in southern France bordering the Mediterranean Sea. This delicate fish dish, flavored with herbs, chopped black olives, extra-virgin olive oil, and white wine encapsulates the flavors of the region. Serve with steamed or boiled potatoes sprinkled with freshly ground pepper and sea salt and drizzled with a little extra-virgin olive oil.

SERVES 4

6 tablespoons extra-virgin olive oil
4 tablespoons white wine
12 pitted black olives, finely chopped
2 cloves garlic, finely chopped
2 tablespoons finely chopped fresh flat-leaf parsley
1 teaspoon Dijon mustard
1 teaspoon sea salt
½ teaspoon fresh ground black pepper
32 green beans, ends trimmed
20 cherry tomatoes, halved
Four 6-ounce (180 g) uncooked whitefish fillets (such as snapper, cod, or haddock)
20 thinly sliced red onion rings

Preheat the oven to 440°F (225°C). In a bowl, mix together the olive oil, white wine, olives, garlic, parsley, mustard, salt, and pepper until well combined. Place a quarter of the green beans and cherry tomatoes in the center of each of four 12-inch pieces of foil. Place a fish fillet on top of each bed of vegetables. Spoon a quarter of the oil mixture over each fillet and arrange the red onion rings on top. Fold the foil over the fish and vegetables and seal the foil packets tightly (fold the edges together so no steam can escape).

Place the packets on a baking sheet and bake in the oven for 16 minutes. Remove the packets from the oven and open (be careful—the steam is very hot). Transfer the fish and vegetables to serving plates and drizzle with the cooking juices.

Rice and Grain Dishes

Shrimp, Tomato, Pea, and Basil Risotto

Risottos are usually quite time-consuming to make because you have to stand over the cooking pot and stir constantly while regularly adding small amounts of stock. In some parts of Italy they've discovered that you don't have to go to such trouble in order to end up with a delicious creamy risotto. By simply adding all the ingredients to the pot, then covering with a lid, the risotto will cook by itself without the need to stir at all. In this risotto, tangy tomatoes and flavorful basil combine exquisitely with shrimp and peas.

SERVES 4

6 tablespoons extra-virgin olive oil
2 onions, finely chopped
4 cloves garlic, finely chopped
2 cups arborio rice
4 ripe tomatoes, diced
1/2 cup frozen green peas, thawed
1 cup white wine
4 cups fish, chicken, or vegetable stock
1 teaspoon sea salt
1/2 teaspoon freshly ground black pepper
32 large uncooked shrimp (prawns), peeled and deveined
2 tablespoons finely chopped fresh basil
2/3 cup grated Parmesan cheese

Heat 4 tablespoons of the olive oil in a large saucepan over medium heat and cook the onions, stirring occasionally, until softened, about 5 minutes. Add the garlic and rice and cook for 1 minute, stirring to coat the rice with oil. Add the tomatoes, peas, wine, stock, salt, and pepper, bring to a boil, cover with a lid, and reduce the heat to low. Simmer gently for 15 minutes without lifting the lid. Remove the lid, quickly place the shrimp on top of the rice, cover, and cook for 5 minutes. Stir the basil, cheese, and reserved olive oil through the rice and serve.

Chicken Risotto with Red Pepper, Arugula, and Olives

The delicate peppery flavor of the arugula and the heat of the chile are highlighted by the sweetness of the red pepper.

SERVES 4

6 tablespoons extra-virgin olive oil
2 onions, finely chopped
4 cloves garlic, finely chopped
2 red bell peppers, finely diced
2 small red chiles, deseeded and finely chopped
2 cups arborio rice
1 cup white wine
4 cups chicken stock
1 teaspoon sea salt
$\frac{1}{2}$ teaspoon freshly ground black pepper
24 ounces (720 g) uncooked skinless chicken breast fillets, cut into bite-size pieces
4 cups arugula (rocket), stems trimmed, and leaves washed and roughly chopped
$\frac{2}{3}$ cup grated Parmesan cheese
16 pitted black olives, sliced

Heat 4 tablespoons of the olive oil in a large saucepan over medium heat and cook the onions, stirring occasionally, until softened, about 5 minutes. Add the garlic, bell peppers, and chiles and cook for 1 minute. Add the rice and cook for another minute, stirring to coat the grains with oil. Add the wine, stock, salt, and pepper, bring to a boil, cover with a lid, and reduce the heat to low. Simmer gently for 12 minutes without lifting the lid. Remove the lid, quickly place the chicken and arugula on top of the rice, cover, and cook for 8 minutes. Stir the cheese, olives, and reserved olive oil through the rice and serve.

Risotto Primavera

Primavera is Italian for spring, and this colorful risotto is a great way of celebrating the arrival of tender spring vegetables.

SERVES 4

½ cup pine nuts
6 tablespoons extra-virgin olive oil
2 onions, finely chopped
4 cloves garlic, finely chopped
2 cups arborio rice
16 fresh asparagus spears, ends trimmed, cut into 1-inch pieces
16 cherry tomatoes, halved
8 white button mushrooms, thickly sliced
½ cup frozen green peas, thawed
1 cup white wine
4 cups vegetable or chicken stock
1 teaspoon sea salt
½ teaspoon freshly ground black pepper
4 tablespoons chopped fresh basil
⅔ cup grated Parmesan cheese

Toast the pine nuts in a large saucepan over medium heat for 1 minute, then set aside.

Heat 4 tablespoons of the olive oil in the same saucepan over medium heat and cook the onions, stirring occasionally, until softened, about 5 minutes. Add the garlic and rice and cook for 1 minute, stirring to coat the grains with oil. Add the asparagus, tomatoes, and mushrooms and cook for another minute. Add the peas, wine, stock, salt, and pepper, bring to a boil, then cover with a lid, and reduce the heat to low. Simmer gently for 20 minutes without lifting the lid. Stir the basil, cheese, pine nuts, and reserved olive oil through the rice and serve.

VARIATIONS: Lots of vegetables work well—green beans, broccoli florets, corn kernels, zucchini, celery, or carrots—choose a variety of colors and textures.

You can also jazz up this risotto by adding some chopped canned artichoke hearts or sun-dried tomatoes.

Mushroom, Bacon, and Walnut Risotto

This rustic risotto is one of our favorites. The mushrooms, walnuts, and creamy arborio rice make a wonderful combination, and the bacon is used in small amounts as a flavor and texture enhancer.

6 tablespoons extra-virgin olive oil
2 onions, finely chopped
4 bacon slices, fat and rind removed, and diced
2 cups arborio rice
14 ounces (400 g) white button mushrooms, cleaned and thickly sliced
4 cloves garlic, finely chopped
$\frac{1}{2}$ cup roughly chopped walnuts
4 cups chicken stock
1 cup white wine
1 teaspoon sea salt
$\frac{1}{2}$ teaspoon freshly ground black pepper
2 tablespoons finely chopped fresh flat-leaf parsley
$\frac{2}{3}$ cup grated Parmesan cheese

Heat 4 tablespoons of the olive oil in a large saucepan over medium heat and cook the onions, stirring occasionally, until softened, about 3 minutes. Add the bacon and cook, stirring regularly, for 2 minutes. Add the rice, mushrooms, garlic, and walnuts and cook, stirring to coat the rice with oil, for 1 minute. Add the stock, wine, salt, and pepper, bring to a boil, cover with a lid, and reduce the heat to low. Simmer gently for 20 minutes without lifting the lid. Stir the parsley, cheese, and reserved olive oil through the rice and serve.

TIP: Replace the regular bacon with soy bacon if you don't eat meat.

Salmon Kedgeree

Kedgeree is based on a traditional Indian rice and lentil dish called *kitchri*, which was adapted by the British to be a breakfast dish containing fish. This hearty kedgeree makes an ideal leisurely weekend breakfast, or it can turn up just as easily on the lunch or dinner table.

SERVES 4

4 teaspoons canola oil
4 teaspoons butter
2 onions, finely chopped
2 carrots, peeled and finely chopped
4 cloves garlic, minced
6 teaspoons good-quality curry powder
1½ cups basmati or long-grain white rice
3 cups fish or vegetable stock
2 teaspoons brown sugar
2 teaspoons salt
4 large eggs
14 ounces (420 g) canned Alaskan red salmon, drained, bones removed,
    broken into chunks
½ cup frozen green peas, thawed
2 tablespoons freshly squeezed lemon juice
2 tablespoons finely chopped cilantro (fresh coriander)

Heat the oil and butter in a large skillet over medium heat and cook the onions and carrots, stirring occasionally, until softened, about 8 minutes. Add the garlic and curry powder and cook, stirring, for 1 minute. Add the rice and cook, stirring to coat the grains, for another minute. Add the stock, sugar, and salt; stir to combine, bring to a boil, and cover with a lid. Reduce the heat to low and simmer gently for 15 minutes without lifting the lid.

While the rice cooks, place the eggs in a pot of boiling water and cook until hard-boiled, about 6 minutes. Remove the eggs from pot, peel, cut into quarters, and set aside.

Remove the skillet lid, quickly place the salmon and peas on top of the rice, replace the lid, and cook for another 5 minutes. Add the lemon juice and cilantro and fluff up the rice gently with a fork to combine the ingredients. Serve the kedgeree on plates with the quartered eggs on top.

VARIATION: Replace the salmon with canned tuna or use sliced smoked salmon for a lavish alternative.

Bulgur Pilaf with Fava Beans, Red Peppers, and Pine Nuts

Bulgur is used in abundance throughout the Middle East—either to accompany stews and casseroles, added to salads, or as a base for a pilaf like this one.

SERVES 4

4 tablespoons pine nuts

4 tablespoons extra-virgin olive oil

2 onions, finely chopped

2 red bell peppers, deseeded and thinly sliced

2 cups frozen fava (broad) beans, thawed, leathery outer skin removed

4 cloves garlic, finely chopped

1 teaspoon dried rosemary

1½ cups bulgur

3 cups chicken stock

2 teaspoons sea salt

1 teaspoon freshly ground black pepper

2 tablespoons chopped fresh flat-leaf parsley

Toast the pine nuts in a large skillet over medium heat for 1 minute, then set aside. Heat 2 tablespoons of the oil in the same skillet over medium heat. Add the onions and bell peppers and cook, stirring occasionally, until softened, about 5 minutes. Add the fava beans, garlic, and rosemary and cook, stirring occasionally, for another 2 minutes. Add the bulgur and cook, stirring, for 1 minute to lightly toast it. Stir in the stock, salt, and pepper, bring to a boil, then cover the skillet with a lid. Reduce the heat to low and let the bulgur steam for 15 minutes. Fluff up the bulgur with a fork, stir in the pine nuts, remaining olive oil, and parsley, and serve.

Tunisian Chicken and Almond Couscous

Couscous, a staple food of North Africa, is one of the most ancient convenience foods and is ready to eat in five minutes. In this dish, couscous is steamed in stock with chicken, vegetables, and spices, becoming light and fluffy as it soaks up the delicious Tunisian-inspired flavors.

SERVES 4

6 tablespoons sliced almonds

6 tablespoons extra-virgin olive oil

24 ounces (720 g) uncooked skinless chicken breast fillets, cut into bite-size pieces

1 red bell pepper, julienned

1 green bell pepper, julienned

2 scallions (white and green parts), trimmed and thinly sliced

4 cloves garlic, finely chopped

2 teaspoons ground cumin

2 teaspoons paprika

2 teaspoons sea salt

1½ teaspoon ground black pepper

1 teaspoon cinnamon

2 cups couscous

4 cups chicken stock

2 tablespoons freshly squeezed lemon juice

4 tablespoons chopped fresh flat-leaf parsley

Toast the almonds in a large skillet over medium heat for 1 minute, then set aside. Heat 4 tablespoons of the oil in the same skillet over medium heat and cook the chicken, stirring occasionally, for about 2 minutes. Add the bell peppers and cook, stirring occasionally, for 4 minutes. Add the scallions, garlic, cumin, paprika, salt, pepper, and cinnamon and cook, stirring, for another minute. Add the couscous and stock, bring to a boil, cover with a lid, then remove the skillet from the heat. Allow to stand for 5 minutes, without lifting the lid, so the couscous absorbs the stock. Fluff up the couscous with a fork; stir in the lemon juice, parsley, reserved olive oil, and almonds; and serve.

SERVING IDEA: This dish can be served with a dollop of plain Greek-style yogurt.

VARIATION: Canned chickpeas (rinsed and drained) are a good alternative to chicken.

Shrimp Fried Rice

A traditional Chinese fried rice dish with fresh succulent shrimp, red pepper, zucchini, and green peas.

SERVES 4

2 cups long-grain white rice
6 tablespoons soy sauce
2 tablespoons oyster sauce
4 teaspoons sesame oil
6 tablespoons peanut oil or canola oil
32 large uncooked shrimp (prawns), peeled and deveined
1 red bell pepper, diced
2 zucchini (courgette), diced
1 cup frozen green peas, thawed
4 cloves garlic, minced

Bring 3 cups of water to a boil in a saucepan. Stir in the rice, and keep stirring until the water returns to a boil. Cover the pot with a tight-fitting lid, reduce the heat to very low, and simmer gently for 15 minutes. Leave the rice to cool (preferably in the fridge overnight).

Mix together the soy sauce, oyster sauce, and sesame oil in a small bowl and set aside.

Heat a wok or large skillet over high heat, then add 2 tablespoons of the peanut oil. Add the shrimp and cook, stirring, for 2 minutes. Remove the shrimp from the wok and set aside on a plate. Heat the remaining 4 tablespoons of oil in the same pan, add the bell peppers, and cook, stirring, for 1 minute. Add the zucchini and cook, stirring, for 2 minutes. Add the peas and garlic and cook, stirring, for 30 seconds. Add the rice and stir for another minute, tossing to separate the grains, and combine well. Add the sauce mixture and cook, stirring, for 2 minutes. Add the cooked shrimp, toss to mix, and heat through, and serve.

Ham and Egg Fried Rice

Ham and eggs not only make a good breakfast combination, they also taste great together in this fried rice dish. In fact, you could even eat this dish as a breakfast.

SERVES 4

2 cups long-grain white rice
6 tablespoons soy sauce
2 tablespoons oyster sauce
2 teaspoons sesame oil
4 tablespoons peanut oil or canola oil
1 red bell pepper, diced
2 zucchini (courgette), diced
1 cup frozen green peas, thawed
4 cloves garlic, minced
4 thin ham slices, finely chopped
4 large eggs

Bring 3 cups of water to a boil in a saucepan. Stir in the rice and keep stirring until the water returns to a boil. Cover the pot with a tight-fitting lid, reduce the heat to very low, and simmer gently for 15 minutes. Leave the rice to cool (preferably in the fridge overnight).

Mix together the soy sauce, oyster sauce, and sesame oil in a small bowl and set aside.

Heat a wok or large skillet over high heat and add the peanut oil. Add the bell pepper and cook, stirring, for 2 minutes. Add the zucchini and cook, stirring, for 2 minutes. Add the peas and garlic and stir for 30 seconds, then add the ham and eggs and stir for another minute. Add the rice and stir, tossing to separate the grains, and combine well, for a minute. Add the sauce mixture; cook, stirring, for 2 minutes and serve.

Noodle Dishes

Seafood Chow Mein

Chow mein is Chinese for "fried noodles." Cooking your own chow mein at home is quick and simple, and it's a great way to use up whatever spare ingredients you have on hand. In this version we combine noodles with fresh seafood, colorful vegetables, and a delicate Chinese-style sauce.

8 ounces (240 g) dried Chinese wheat noodles
4 tablespoons soy sauce
2 tablespoons black bean sauce
4 tablespoons oyster sauce
2 tablespoons Chinese rice wine (or dry sherry)
1 tablespoon brown sugar
6 tablespoons canola or peanut oil
12 large uncooked shrimp (prawns), peeled and deveined
12 uncooked large scallops
2 squid tubes, cut into bite-size pieces
2 red bell peppers, julienned
20 snow peas, ends trimmed, cut in half on the diagonal
2 bunches bok choy or choy sum, washed and roughly chopped
4 cloves garlic, minced
4 teaspoons finely grated fresh ginger

Add the dried noodles to a saucepan of boiling water and cook for 5 minutes, then rinse under cold water and set aside.

Mix together the soy sauce, black bean sauce, oyster sauce, Chinese rice wine, and sugar in a bowl and set aside.

Heat a wok or large skillet over high heat, add 2 tablespoons of the oil and cook the shrimp and scallops, stirring, for 1½ minutes. Add the squid and cook, stirring, for 1 minute, then remove the seafood from the wok and set aside on a plate.

Add the remaining oil to the wok and cook the bell peppers, stirring, for 3 minutes. Add the snow peas and bok choy or choy sum and cook, stirring, for another 4 minutes. Add the garlic and ginger, stir for 1 minute, then return the seafood to the wok. Add the noodles to the wok and stir to combine. Add the sauce mixture and cook, stirring, for 1 minute until thoroughly combined, and serve.

Chicken and Ham Chow Mein in Peking Sauce

An assortment of crisp vegetables, chicken, and ham are tossed with soft noodles in a delicate Peking-style sauce.

SERVES 4

8 ounces (240 g) dried Chinese wheat noodles
4 tablespoons soy sauce
6 tablespoons hoisin sauce
2 tablespoons Chinese rice wine (or dry sherry)
2 teaspoons sesame oil
4 tablespoons canola or peanut oil
12 ounces (360 g) uncooked skinless chicken breast fillet, cut into bite-size pieces
2 carrots, peeled and julienned
2 cups broccoli florets
4 cups shredded Chinese (Napa) cabbage
4 thin ham slices, chopped
4 cloves garlic, minced
1 tablespoon finely grated fresh ginger
2 scallions (white and green parts), trimmed and thinly sliced

Add the dried noodles to a saucepan of boiling water and cook for 5 minutes, then rinse under cold water and set aside.

Mix together the soy sauce, hoisin sauce, Chinese rice wine, and sesame oil in a bowl and set aside.

Heat a wok or large skillet over high heat, add 2 tablespoons of the canola oil, and cook the chicken, stirring, for 4 minutes. Remove the chicken from the wok and set aside on a plate.

Add the remaining canola oil to the wok and cook the carrots and broccoli, stirring, for 4 minutes. Add the cabbage and cook, stirring, for another 2 minutes. Add the ham, garlic, and ginger, stir for 1 minute, then return the chicken to the wok. Add the noodles and stir to combine. Add the sauce mixture and scallions, mix to heat through, and serve.

VARIATION: Replace the chicken and ham with tofu, shrimp, or scallops; add other vegetables like green beans, snow peas, red and green bell peppers, or mushrooms (fresh or dried).

Tofu and Cashew Chow Mein

Crunchy cashews and vegetables complement the soft texture of the noodles and tofu in this quick and satisfying dish.

SERVES 4

20 ounces (600 g) precooked thick Chinese wheat noodles (typically found
   in the refrigerated section of the supermarket)
6 tablespoons soy sauce
4 tablespoons oyster sauce
4 teaspoons sesame oil
4 tablespoons water
4 tablespoons canola or peanut oil
2 carrots, peeled and julienned
4 cups small broccoli florets
12 ounces (360 g) firm tofu, cut into cubes
4 cloves garlic, minced
4 teaspoons finely grated fresh ginger
1 cup roasted cashew nuts

Loosen the precooked noodles by soaking in a bowl of hot water for 2 to 3 minutes, then drain and set aside.

Mix together the soy sauce, oyster sauce, sesame oil, and water in a bowl and set aside.

Heat a wok or large skillet over high heat, add the canola oil, and cook the carrots and broccoli, stirring, for 2 minutes. Add the tofu and cook, stirring, for 4 minutes. Add the garlic and ginger and stir for 1 minute. Add the noodles and stir to combine. Add the sauce mixture and cashews, mix until thoroughly combined and heated through, and serve.

VARIATION: Replace the cashews with sliced almonds.

Teriyaki Chicken Noodles

The savory-sweet teriyaki sauce combines perfectly with the tender chicken and vegetables in this quick and flavorful noodle dish.

SERVES 4

7 ounces (200 g) dried somen noodles
½ cup water
8 tablespoons soy sauce
6 tablespoons mirin (rice wine)
4 teaspoons brown sugar
4 tablespoons peanut or canola oil
24 ounces (720 g) uncooked skinless chicken breast fillets, cut into bite-size pieces
2 carrots, peeled and julienned
Small bunch of bok choy, washed and roughly chopped
4 teaspoons finely grated fresh ginger
2 scallions (white and green parts), trimmed and finely sliced on the diagonal
4 teaspoons cornstarch (corn flour), mixed to a paste with 4 teaspoons water

Cook the noodles in a pot of boiling water for 3 minutes, then drain under cold water and set aside.

Mix together the water, soy sauce, mirin, and brown sugar in a bowl and set aside.

Heat a wok or large skillet over high heat, add 2 tablespoons of the oil, and cook the chicken, stirring, for 5 minutes. Remove the chicken from the pan and set aside on a plate.

Scrape the wok or skillet clean. Add the remaining oil and cook the carrots and bok choy, stirring, until softened, for 7 minutes. Add the cooked somen noodles and stir for 30 seconds. Add the ginger, scallions, and chicken and cook, stirring, for 1 minute. Add the sauce and stir to combine. While stirring constantly, add the cornstarch paste, cook until the sauce thickens, and serve.

VARIATION: This dish can easily be transformed into Teriyaki Scallop Noodles by replacing the chicken with 24 ounces (720 g) of uncooked large scallops, which you need to stir-fry for only 2 minutes.

Malaysian Fish Laksa

A traditional Malaysian *laksa* (noodle soup) with tender fish pieces, rice noodles, vegetables, and a variety of authentic spices and seasonings.

SERVES 4

4 tablespoons peanut or canola oil

2 onions, finely chopped

4 cloves garlic, finely chopped

4 teaspoons finely grated fresh ginger

2 teaspoons finely grated lemon zest

1 teaspoon shrimp paste (or 2 tablespoons fish sauce added with
   the stock and coconut milk)

5 cups chicken stock

3 cups coconut milk

2 tablespoons freshly squeezed lemon juice

3 teaspoons turmeric

1 teaspoon ground coriander

2 teaspoons *sambal oelek*, or 1 teaspoon chili powder

2 teaspoons brown sugar

2 teaspoons salt

7 ounces (200 g) rice stick noodles (or, if available, use laksa noodles)

24 ounces (720 g) firm oily fish fillets (such as mackerel or swordfish),
   cut into bite-size pieces

2 cups bean sprouts

A handful of cilantro (fresh coriander), stems removed

2 scallions (white and green parts), trimmed and thinly sliced on the diagonal

2 small fresh red chiles, finely diced

Heat the oil in a large saucepan over a medium heat. Add the onions and cook, stirring, for 2 minutes. Add the garlic and cook, stirring occasionally, for 3 minutes. Add the ginger, lemon zest, and shrimp paste and cook, stirring to dissolve the shrimp paste, for a minute. Add the stock, coconut milk, lemon juice, turmeric, coriander, sambal oelek, sugar, and salt, stir to combine, and bring to a boil. Reduce the heat to reach a rolling simmer and cook for 6 minutes.

While the laksa simmers, soak the noodles in boiling water for 10 minutes.

Add the fish pieces to the laksa and cook another 4 minutes. Drain the noodles and place equal amounts in bowls. Top with equal amounts of bean sprouts, cilantro, scallions, and chiles. Ladle the laksa over the top and serve immediately.

Japanese Tuna and Vegetable Udon Noodle Pot

In this one-pot meal, tuna and vegetables are simmered in a flavorsome stock, then served over soft and slippery udon noodles.

SERVES 4

4 ounces (120 g) dried udon noodles
8 cups chicken stock
24 ounces (720 g) fresh tuna steak, cut into bite-size pieces
4 cups shredded green cabbage
2 carrots, peeled and julienned
20 snow peas, ends trimmed and cut in half on the diagonal
16 fresh shiitake mushrooms, stems removed and sliced into halves
2 teaspoons finely grated fresh ginger
4 tablespoons Japanese soy sauce
2 tablespoons freshly squeezed lemon juice
2 scallions (white and green parts), trimmed and thinly sliced

Add the dried udon noodles to a saucepan of boiling water and cook for 7 minutes.

Place the stock in a large saucepan and bring to a boil. Add the tuna, cabbage, carrots, snow peas, mushrooms, and ginger and return to a boil. Cover the pot, reduce the heat, and simmer for 7 minutes. Remove from the heat and stir in the soy sauce and lemon juice. Drain the noodles and put equal amounts into soup bowls and scatter scallions on top. Pour the boiling tuna–vegetable broth over to cover and allow to stand for 1 minute. Serve with chopsticks and a soup spoon.

VARIATIONS: Replace the tuna with chicken, shrimp, or scallops.

Cubes of firm tofu also make a tasty addition (tofu soaks up flavors well).

Dried rice or cellophane noodles that have been soaked until soft can replace the udon noodles. You can use dried shiitake mushrooms instead of fresh ones; however, you'll need to rehydrate them before use.

Peanut Chicken Noodles

Long, slippery rice noodles with strips of stir-fried chicken and vegetables in a rich and spicy Indonesian peanut sauce.

SERVES 4

10 ounces (300 g) dried rice stick noodles
4 tablespoons peanut or canola oil
24 ounces (720 g) uncooked skinless chicken breast fillets, cut into strips
2 carrots, peeled and julienned
2 zucchini, julienned
2 cups Indonesian Peanut Sauce (page 282), hot

Soak the rice stick noodles in boiling water for 10 minutes, then rinse under cold water and set aside.

Heat a wok or large skillet over high heat then add 2 tablespoons of the oil. Cook the chicken, stirring, for 3 minutes, then remove from the wok and set aside on a plate.

Add the remaining oil to the hot wok and cook the carrots, stirring, for 1 minute. Add the zucchini and cook, stirring, for another 3 minutes. Add the cooked noodles and chicken and toss to combine and heat through. Pour in the hot peanut sauce, thoroughly mix all the ingredients together, and serve.

VARIATIONS: Shrimp (prawns), scallops, or tofu can replace the chicken. Replace the carrots with julienned red bell peppers.

Asian Cilantro-Peanut Pesto Noodles with Chicken, Broccoli, and Red Pepper

This recipe combines rice noodles with chicken, lightly steamed vegetables, and an Asian-inspired pesto.

SERVES 4

8 ounces (240 g) dried rice stick noodles
2 red bell peppers, julienned

4 cups broccoli florets
1½ cups Asian Cilantro-Peanut Pesto (page 260)
24 ounces (720 g) cooked skinless chicken breast, shredded

Soak the noodles in boiling water for 10 minutes.

While the noodles are soaking, steam the red peppers and broccoli in a steamer pan for 6 minutes. Drain the noodles, toss with the pesto, steamed vegetables, and chicken until thoroughly combined and serve.

VARIATION: Replace the chicken with cooked seafood or cubes of firm tofu.

Soba Noodle Scallops

This delicate Japanese broth with soba noodles and tender scallops is simple to prepare and highly satisfying.

SERVES 4

8 cups *dashi* stock (dashi stock powder is available at Asian food stores)
4 tablespoons soy sauce
2 carrots, peeled and julienned
4 teaspoons finely grated fresh ginger
6 ounces (180 g) thin soba noodles
24 uncooked large scallops
2 scallions (white and green parts), trimmed and thinly sliced on the diagonal

Bring 8 cups of dashi stock to a boil in a saucepan. Add the soy sauce, carrots, and ginger and simmer, covered, for 6 minutes.

While the broth simmers, cook the noodles in boiling water in a separate saucepan for 4 minutes, then drain.

Add the scallops to the broth, simmer for 2 minutes, remove from the heat, and add the noodles. Serve in bowls with scallions scattered on top.

VARIATIONS: Use large, peeled raw shrimp instead of the scallops. Add some sliced fresh white button mushrooms.

Mie Goreng (Indonesian Fried Noodles)

An Indonesian fried noodle dish with shrimp, pork, and vegetables, flavored with a spicy sauce mixture, and topped with fresh cilantro and crisp cucumber.

SERVES 4

8 ounces (240 g) dried Chinese wheat noodles
4 tablespoons soy sauce
4 tablespoons *kecap manis* (Indonesian sweet soy sauce, which is available
  at Asian food stores)
3 tablespoons fish sauce
2 teaspoons *sambal oelek* (Indonesian chile sauce)
4 tablespoons peanut oil or canola
10 ounces (300 g) lean pork, finely diced
4 cups shredded green cabbage
4 scallions (white and green parts), trimmed and thinly sliced
6 cloves garlic, crushed
10 ounces (300 g) small peeled cooked shrimp
Finely chopped cilantro (fresh coriander), for garnish
Thin strips of cucumber, for garnish

Add the dried noodles to a saucepan of boiling water and cook for 5 minutes, then rinse under cold water and set aside.

Mix together the soy sauce, kecap manis, fish sauce, and sambal oelek in a bowl and set aside.

Heat the oil in a wok or large skillet over high heat and cook the pork, stirring, for 3 minutes. Add the cabbage and cook, stirring, for 2 minutes. Add the scallions and garlic and cook, stirring, for 2 minutes. Add the noodles, shrimp, and sauce mixture and stir for 1 minute to combine well and heat through. Serve in bowls garnished with cilantro and cucumber strips on top.

VARIATION: Replace the pork with lean bacon or ham.

Sushi and Rice Paper Rolls

▶ Sushi Rolls

There are two main types of sushi, *nigiri-zushi*, which is vinegared rice, hand-formed into oval shapes and topped with various raw and cooked seafood, and *maki-zushi*, which is vinegared rice, combined with seafood and vegetables then wrapped in an edible seaweed called nori and sliced into rounds. Nigiri-zushi is quite finicky to make at home, and we tend to eat this type of sushi at Japanese restaurants and sushi bars. Maki-zushi, on the other hand, is far easier to prepare in your own kitchen, and the taste of these delightful morsels has left many (including us) with an addiction for life! This sushi recipe requires a sushi mat for rolling.

SERVES 4

2½ cups Japanese short-grain white rice (like Koshihikari rice)
2½ cups cold water
4 tablespoons rice vinegar
3 tablespoons sugar
2 teaspoons salt
Your choice of fillings (Sushi Roll Variations, page 208)
6 sheets nori
Wasabi paste, for serving
Japanese soy sauce, for serving
Pickled ginger (*gari*), for serving

Place the rice in a colander and rinse thoroughly under the tap until the water runs clear, then drain well. Place the rice and the cold water in a medium saucepan and bring to a boil. Cover the saucepan, turn the heat down to very low, and cook for 15 minutes without lifting the lid. Turn off the heat, allow to stand for 10 minutes, still covered, then spoon the rice into a large bowl.

Mix together the vinegar, sugar, and salt in a small bowl until the sugar dissolves, then drizzle over the rice. Mix together gently to coat the rice with the sushi vinegar, then set aside to cool to room temperature. Toast each nori sheet very lightly by passing back and forth quickly over a stove-top burner (don't place it too close to the heat or else the delicate nori will burn). To fill and roll the sushi rolls, see the diagram opposite.

▶ Spread the cooked rice over the nori sheet.

▶ Smear a small amount of wasabi in a line across the middle of the rice (be sparing with wasabi, it's hot!).

▶ Arrange small portions of your chosen fillings on top of the wasabi in a horizontal line down the center of the rice.

▶ Roll up the sushi tightly with the sushi mat to form a neatly packed cylinder (like a fat cigar).

▶ Squeeze firmly to make sure the sushi roll is tightly packed (be careful not to squeeze too hard or you'll break the sushi roll).

continues on next page

6

▶ Cut each sushi roll into 1½-inch rounds using a sharp, damp knife (it's important that you remoisten the knife after each cut).

7

▶ Serve the sushi with a small bowl of shoyu (soy sauce) for dipping, extra wasabi for those who like their sushi extra hot, and slices of gari (Japanese pickled ginger) for cleansing the palate between sushi pieces.

VARIATIONS: The range of possible fillings for sushi rolls is enormous. By mixing and matching various ingredients you can create many different varieties. Here are some popular sushi roll fillings:

SMOKED SALMON	CUCUMBER
COOKED SHRIMP (PRAWNS)	AVOCADO
CRAB (OR SURIMI)	SCALLIONS
VERY FRESH RAW TUNA AND SALMON	MUSHROOMS
TOFU (FIRM OR SILKEN)	SNOW PEAS
EGGS (MADE INTO AN OMELET	SNOW PEA SPROUTS
AND CUT INTO STRIPS)	ASPARAGUS (LIGHTLY STEAMED)
TOASTED SESAME SEEDS	CARROT

Our Favorite Sushi Rolls

Each of the following sushi recipes makes 6 sushi rolls (or approximately 36 sushi rounds):

SMOKED SALMON AND AVOCADO SUSHI ROLLS

Cut 6 ounces (180 g) of sliced smoked salmon into thin strips. Peel an avocado and cut the flesh into strips. Smear a small amount of wasabi in a horizontal line across the middle of each rice-topped nori sheet and arrange equal amounts of salmon and avocado on top. Roll the sushi up and cut into 1½-inch rounds to serve.

TUNA AND CUCUMBER SUSHI ROLLS

Cut a 10-ounce (300 g) piece of very fresh raw tuna into thin strips. Peel and remove the seeds from half a small cucumber and cut the flesh into thin strips. Smear a small amount of wasabi in a horizontal line across the middle of each rice-topped nori sheet and arrange equal amounts of tuna and cucumber on top. Roll the sushi up and cut into 1½-inch rounds to serve.

SHRIMP AND VEGETABLE SUSHI ROLLS

Cut 12 large peeled, cooked shrimp (prawns) in half lengthways. Peel and remove the seeds from half a small cucumber and cut the flesh into thin strips. Trim and cut 2 scallions (white and green parts) into thin diagonal slices and thinly slice the flesh of ½ avocado. Smear a small amount of wasabi in a horizontal line across the middle of each rice-topped nori sheet and arrange equal amounts of each filling on top. Roll the sushi up and cut into 1½-inch rounds to serve.

TOFU, SESAME, AND MIXED VEGETABLE SUSHI ROLLS

Lightly toast 3 teaspoons of sesame seeds in a frying pan. Cut 7 ounces (200 g) of firm tofu into thin strips. Peel and grate a small carrot. Remove the stems from 6 fresh shitake mushrooms (or use soaked, dried mushrooms or regular mushrooms) and thinly slice. Wash and drain ½ cup snow pea sprouts. Smear a small amount of wasabi in a horizontal line across the middle of each rice-topped nori sheet and arrange equal quantities of each filling on top. Roll the sushi up and cut into 1½-inch rounds to serve.

continues on next page

► CALIFORNIA SUSHI ROLLS

Cut 10 ounces (300 g) of crab (or imitation crab, surimi) into thin strips and mix with 2 tablespoons of Japanese or regular mayonnaise. Peel an avocado and cut the flesh into strips. Peel and remove the seeds from half a small cucumber and cut the flesh into thin strips. Smear a small amount of wasabi in a horizontal line across the middle of each rice-topped nori sheet and arrange equal amounts of crab, cucumber, and avocado on top. Roll the sushi up and cut into 1½-inch rounds to serve. As a variation, replace the crab with cooked shrimp.

► EGG AND VEGETABLE SUSHI ROLLS

Cook an ordinary omelet using 2 eggs seasoned with salt and pepper, then slice it into thin strips. Cut 12 snow peas into thin strips and grate a small carrot. Smear a small amount of wasabi in a horizontal line across the middle of each rice-topped nori sheet and arrange equal amounts of each filling on top. Roll the sushi up and cut into 1½-inch rounds to serve.

► SMOKED SALMON AND ASPARAGUS SUSHI ROLLS

Cut 6 ounces (180 g) of sliced smoked salmon into strips. Lightly steam 12 trimmed asparagus spears, then cool them in cold water. Smear a small amount of wasabi in a horizontal line across the middle of each rice-topped nori sheet and arrange equal amounts of salmon and asparagus on top. Roll the sushi up and cut into 1½-inch rounds to serve.

Rice Paper Rolls

These soft, uncooked rolls—which are popular in Vietnam and parts of China—make a refreshing change to deep-fried spring rolls. Nutritious fillings including noodles, seafood, chicken, fresh vegetables, and aromatic herbs are wrapped in delicate rice paper sheets and served cold with the dipping sauces of your choice. You can prepare these rolls up to 4 hours ahead and chill them in the refrigerator, covered with a clean dampened dish towel to keep them moist, until you're ready to serve.

These rolls can also be panfried. Heat 2 tablespoons of canola oil in a large frying pan until hot. Panfry 4 rice paper rolls at a time for a total of 9 minutes, turning each roll every 3 minutes so they are golden and crisp all over. Repeat the cooking process with the remaining rolls.

SERVES 4

1 ounce (30 g) dried rice vermicelli noodles
1 tablespoon rice vinegar
1 tablespoon water
1 teaspoon sugar
$\frac{1}{2}$ teaspoon salt
1 clove garlic, minced
Your choice of fillings (Rice Paper Roll Variations follow)
8 rice paper sheets
Your choice of Nuoc Cham Dipping Sauce (page 284), Chinese-Style Dipping
    Sauce (page 288), Sesame-Hoisin Dipping Sauce (page 288), or sweet chili
    sauce, for serving

Prepare the noodles by placing them in a large bowl and pouring boiling water over them to cover. Let soak until noodles soften and separate when stirred, about 5 minutes.

While the noodles are soaking, mix together the vinegar, water, sugar, salt, and garlic in a small bowl until the sugar dissolves.

Rinse the noodles under cold water, drain well, then cut into 3-inch lengths. Mix together the noodles and the dressing gently to coat. Mix together the dressed noodles with your choice of filling ingredients in a bowl until well combined.

To fill and roll the rice paper rolls, see the diagram on the following page.

HOW TO ROLL RICE PAPER ROLLS

▶ Soak a sheet of rice paper in a large shallow dish of hot water for about 15-20 seconds, then drain well.

▶ Delicately place the sheet of rice paper out on top of a clean dry dishcloth, then place the filling ingredients toward the lower edge of the rice paper.

▶ Neatly fold the bottom edge of the rice paper over the filling.

▶ Fold in the side edges of the rice paper.

▶ Roll up the rice paper roll to form a neatly packed cylinder (like a fat cigar).

▶ Arrange the rice paper rolls on a plate with Nuoc Cham Dipping Sauce (page 284) to serve.

VARIATIONS: There are lots of fillings you can wrap in rice paper sheets. Feel free to come up with your own varieties or use the following suggestions. Here are some popular rice paper roll fillings.

CHICKEN BREAST

COOKED SALMON AND TUNA

COOKED SHRIMP

CRAB (OR SURIMI)

TOFU (FIRM OR SILKEN)

BEAN SPROUTS

RED AND GREEN BELL PEPPERS

CHINESE CABBAGE

CUCUMBER

SCALLIONS

MUSHROOMS

SNOW PEAS

ZUCCHINI

CARROT

WATER CHESTNUTS

MINT

CILANTRO (FRESH CORIANDER)

BASIL

GARLIC

CHILE

GINGER

ROASTED PEANUTS

TOASTED SESAME SEEDS

Our Favorite Rice Paper Rolls

Each of the following variations makes 8 rice paper rolls.

▶ VIETNAMESE SHRIMP AND VEGETABLE ROLLS

Mix together the dressed noodles with ½ cup bean sprouts, 1 peeled and grated carrot, ½ cup finely diced red bell pepper, ½ cup finely diced cucumber, 2 tablespoons of finely chopped fresh mint, 12 ounces (360 g) cooked peeled shrimp, and 2 tablespoons chopped roasted peanuts in a bowl until well combined. Roll up in rice paper sheets and serve with the dipping sauces of your choice—Nuoc Cham Dipping Sauce (page 284) or sweet chili sauce are ideal with these rolls.

▶ CHINESE-STYLE CHICKEN AND VEGETABLE ROLLS

Mix together the dressed noodles with 1 peeled and grated carrot, 8 thinly sliced snow peas, ½ cup finely chopped canned water chestnuts (rinsed and drained), 1 teaspoon finely grated fresh ginger, 2 trimmed and finely sliced scallions (white and green parts), 2 tablespoons finely chopped cilantro (fresh coriander), and 12 ounces (360 g) shredded cooked skinless chicken breast in a bowl until well combined. Roll up in rice paper sheets and serve with the dipping sauces of your choice—Chinese-Style Dipping Sauce (page 288) is particularly good with these rolls.

continues on next page

▶ COMBINATION SEAFOOD ROLLS

Mix together the dressed noodles with 1 cup finely shredded Chinese (Napa) cabbage, ½ cup finely chopped red bell pepper, 1 teaspoon finely grated fresh ginger, 2 tablespoons finely chopped cilantro (fresh coriander), and 6 ounces (180 g) each of shredded crab (or imitation crab, surimi) and cooked shrimp in a bowl until well combined. Roll up in rice paper sheets and serve with the dipping sauces of your choice—these rolls are ideal with Sesame-Hoisin Dipping Sauce (page 288).

▶ MUSHROOM, TOFU, AND SESAME ROLLS

Mix together the dressed noodles with 1 cup finely diced mushrooms, 1 cup cubed tofu, 1 peeled and grated carrot, 2 trimmed and thinly sliced scallions (white and green parts), and 2 tablespoons of lightly toasted sesame seeds in a bowl until well combined. Roll up in rice paper sheets and serve with the dipping sauces of your choice—these rolls are particularly good with Chinese-Style Dipping Sauce (page 288).

▶ FRESH TUNA AND VEGETABLE ROLLS

Cut 12 ounces (360 g) of raw tuna into 3-inch strips. Poach the tuna in simmering water for 4 minutes and set aside to cool. Mix the dressed noodles with 1 cup shredded Chinese (Napa) cabbage, 1 peeled and grated carrot, ½ stick finely chopped celery, 2 trimmed and thinly sliced scallions (white and green parts), 1 teaspoon finely grated fresh ginger, and the cooled poached tuna in a bowl until well combined. Roll up in the rice paper sheets and serve with the dipping sauces of your choice—Chinese-Style Dipping Sauce (page 288) and Sesame-Hoisin Dipping Sauce (page 288) are ideal with these rolls. Good-quality canned tuna (rinsed and drained) makes a reasonable substitute for fresh.

▶ THAI CHICKEN AND BASIL RICE PAPER ROLLS

Mix together the dressed noodles with ½ cup finely diced red bell pepper, ½ cup finely diced zucchini, 1 small seeded and finely chopped red chile, 2 tablespoons finely chopped fresh basil, and 12 ounces (360 g) shredded cooked skinless chicken breast in a bowl until well combined. Roll up in rice paper sheets and serve with the dipping sauces of your choice—sweet chili sauce or Nuoc Cham Dipping Sauce (page 284) are particularly good with these rolls.

Grilled Dishes

Japanese-Style Marinated Grilled Tuna

Fish like tuna and swordfish are ideal for barbecuing because they have a firm and "meaty" texture. These tuna fillets are marinated and basted with a mouthwatering combination of Japanese flavors.

SERVES 4

4 teaspoons finely grated fresh ginger
4 tablespoons Japanese soy sauce
2 tablespoons mirin (rice wine)
2 teaspoons sesame oil
Four 6-ounce (180 g) uncooked tuna steaks

Mix together the ginger, soy sauce, mirin, and sesame oil in a bowl until well combined. Marinate the tuna in the mixture, covered, in the refrigerator for at least 30 minutes.

Cook the fish on a hot grill for 3 minutes on each side, brushing with the marinade, and serve immediately.

SERVING IDEA: This dish is ideal served on a bed of Japanese Soba Noodle Salad (page 252).

Grilled Tuscan Chicken with Asparagus and Red Pepper

This is a great way to enjoy chicken, asparagus, and red pepper—marinated in a blend of olive oil, lemon juice, garlic, oregano, and rosemary and grilled until tender and served with a green salad and crusty bread.

SERVES 4

6 tablespoons extra-virgin olive oil
4 tablespoons freshly squeezed lemon juice
4 cloves garlic, minced
1 teaspoon dried oregano
½ teaspoon dried rosemary
1 teaspoon sea salt
½ teaspoon freshly ground black pepper

Four 6-ounce (180 g) uncooked skinless chicken breast fillets
2 red bell peppers, deseeded and cut into quarters lengthways
16 fresh asparagus spears, bottoms trimmed

Mix together the oil, lemon juice, garlic, oregano, rosemary, salt, and pepper in a bowl until well combined. Marinate the chicken, bell peppers, and asparagus in the mixture, covered, in the refrigerator for at least 30 minutes.

Cook the chicken on a hot grill for 4 minutes on each side, brushing with the marinade. Cook the vegetables on the grill at the same time, turning and brushing regularly with the marinade. Serve immediately.

▶ Marinated Mixed Seafood Grill

There's something very special about the taste of freshly grilled seafood like shrimp, squid, and scallops. This simple olive oil and white wine marinade adds flavor and depth, and also helps keep the seafood tender as it cooks.

SERVES 4

6 tablespoons extra-virgin olive oil
6 tablespoons white wine
2 cloves garlic, minced
2 tablespoons finely chopped fresh flat-leaf parsley
1 teaspoon freshly grated lemon zest
1 teaspoon sea salt
1/2 teaspoon freshly ground black pepper
1/2 teaspoon dried rosemary
10 ounces (300 g) uncooked shrimp, peeled
10 ounces (300 g) uncooked scallops
10 ounces (300 g) uncooked squid, cut into rings or bite-size pieces
Lemon wedges, for serving

Mix together the oil, white wine, garlic, parsley, lemon zest, salt, pepper, and rosemary in a bowl until well combined. Marinate the shrimp, scallops, and squid in the mixture, covered, in the refrigerator for at least 30 minutes.

Cook the shrimp and scallops on a hot grill for 3 minutes, turning and brushing regularly with the marinade. Add the squid and cook for 1 minute more, turning once. Serve immediately with lemon wedges for squeezing.

Mediterranean-Style Grilled Marinated Salmon

Serve these simple and stylish salmon steaks with a crisp salad and fresh crusty bread.

SERVES 4

5 tablespoons extra-virgin olive oil
3 tablespoons freshly squeezed lemon juice
2 tablespoons finely chopped fresh flat-leaf parsley
2 tablespoons finely chopped fresh basil
1 teaspoon sea salt
¼ teaspoon freshly ground black pepper
Four 6-ounce (180 g) uncooked salmon steaks
Lemon wedges, for serving

Mix together the olive oil, lemon juice, parsley, basil, salt, and pepper in a bowl until well combined. Marinate the salmon steaks in the mixture, covered, in the refrigerator for at least 30 minutes.

Cook the salmon on a hot grill for 3 minutes on each side, brushing with the marinade. Serve the salmon with lemon wedges for squeezing.

VARIATION: Use other firm-fleshed fish such as tuna or swordfish in place of the salmon.

TIP: Make sure the cooking surface is really hot so the fish can sear quickly and seal in the juices to keep it deliciously moist on the inside.

Grilled Sweet Chili Scallops

These succulent scallops are coated in a flavorful Thai-inspired marinade and seared quickly on a hot grill so they stay plump and tender.

SERVES 4

4 tablespoons sweet chili sauce
2 tablespoons peanut or canola oil
2 tablespoons fish sauce
2 tablespoons freshly squeezed lemon or lime juice
2 tablespoons finely chopped fresh basil
2 cloves garlic, minced

1 teaspoon salt
24 large uncooked scallops
8 bamboo or wooden skewers, soaked in cold water for 15 minutes to prevent burning

Mix together the chili sauce, oil, fish sauce, lemon or lime juice, basil, garlic, and salt in a small bowl. Marinate the scallops in the mixture, covered, in the refrigerator for at least 30 minutes. Thread the scallops evenly onto each skewer.

Grill the scallops on a hot grill for 1 minute on each side, brushing with the marinade. Remove the scallops from the skewers and serve immediately.

▶ Fresh Tuna and Vegetable Skewers

Fresh tuna is threaded onto skewers with cherry tomatoes, zucchini, red onion, green bell pepper, then marinated in a Mediterranean-style dressing and grilled until tender.

SERVES 4

20 bamboo or wooden skewers, soaked in cold water for 15 minutes to prevent burning
28 ounces (840 g) fresh tuna, cut into 60 even-size cubes
40 cherry tomatoes
4 zucchini (courgettes), cut into ½-inch rounds
2 red onions, cut into wedges
2 green bell peppers, cut into 1½-inch squares
8 tablespoons extra-virgin olive oil
4 tablespoons freshly squeezed lemon juice
4 tablespoons finely chopped fresh flat-leaf parsley
4 cloves garlic, minced
2 teaspoons sea salt
1 teaspoon fresh ground black pepper
Lemon wedges, for serving

Thread the tuna, cherry tomatoes, zucchini, red onions, and bell peppers alternately onto each skewer. Mix together the oil, lemon juice, parsley, garlic, salt, and pepper in a small bowl until well combined and pour over the prepared tuna and vegetable skewers. Marinate, covered, in the refrigerator for 1 hour, turning the skewers halfway through marinating time.

Cook the skewers on a hot grill for 12 minutes, turning and brushing regularly with the marinade. Serve the skewers with lemon wedges for squeezing.

Asian Shrimp and Vegetable Skewers

A selection of Asian-style vegetables and shrimp are threaded onto skewers, marinated, and grilled until melt-in-the-mouth tender.

SERVES 4

2 cloves garlic, minced
4 tablespoons canola or peanut oil
6 tablespoons soy sauce
3 tablespoons freshly squeezed lemon juice
4 teaspoons brown sugar
12 bamboo or wooden skewers, soaked in cold water for 15 minutes
    to prevent burning
2 dozen large uncooked shrimp (prawns), peeled
16 fresh mushrooms, cut in half
16 snow peas, ends trimmed and cut in half on the diagonal
2 red bell peppers, cut into small pieces
2 tablespoons finely chopped cilantro (fresh coriander)
Lemon wedges, to serve

Mix together the garlic, oil, soy sauce, lemon juice, and brown sugar in a bowl until well combined. Thread, alternating shrimp, mushrooms, snow peas, and bell peppers, onto the skewers; then marinate them in the mixture, covered, in the refrigerator for at least 20 minutes.

Cook the skewers on a hot grill for 10 to 12 minutes, turning and brushing regularly with the marinade. Sprinkle with the cilantro and serve with lemon wedges for squeezing.

SERVING IDEA: These skewers go perfectly with fried rice.

VARIATION: You can replace the shrimp with scallops, or use a combination of shrimp and scallops.

Thai Fish Parcels

Fish and peppers are cooked in parcels with a simple infusion of Thai flavors.

2 tablespoons finely chopped cilantro (fresh coriander)

2 cloves garlic, minced

2 small red chiles, deseeded and finely chopped

2 teaspoons finely chopped lemongrass or lemon zest

2 teaspoons brown sugar

4 tablespoons fish sauce

2 tablespoons freshly squeezed lime juice

Four 6-ounce (180 g) uncooked firm whitefish fillets (such as snapper, cod, or haddock)

2 red bell peppers, julienned

2 green bell peppers, julienned

Mix together the cilantro, garlic, chiles, lemongrass or zest, sugar, fish sauce, and lime juice in a small bowl. Place each fish fillet in the center of a 12-inch piece of foil and spoon equal amounts of the dressing over each. Arrange the bell peppers on top of the fish. Fold the foil over the fish and vegetables and seal the parcels tightly.

Cook the parcels on a hot grill, on one side only, for 12 minutes. Transfer the fish, vegetables, and sauce from the foil packets to serving plates.

VARIATION: Use skinless chicken breast fillets (and cook for 15 minutes) or seafood such as scallops or shrimp in place of the fish.

Mediterranean-Style Grilled Vegetables

These grilled vegetables are so simple to prepare yet taste absolutely wonderful. Adjust the amount of marinade and vegetables used to the number of mouths to feed.

SERVES 4

6 tablespoons extra-virgin olive oil
3 tablespoons balsamic vinegar
4 cloves garlic, minced
1 teaspoon dried oregano
1 teaspoon dried rosemary
1 teaspoon sea salt
$\frac{1}{2}$ teaspoon freshly ground black pepper

VEGETABLES FOR THE GRILL (CHOOSE ABOUT 8 CUPS OF ANY COMBINATION)
Asparagus, bottoms trimmed, left whole
Mushrooms, peeled or wiped clean, stems removed, caps left whole
    (button mushrooms or portobellos)
Tomatoes, sliced thickly, or whole cherry tomatoes
Red, green, and yellow bell peppers, sliced into strips
Zucchini, cut in half lengthways
Eggplant, cut into $\frac{1}{4}$-inch rounds
Onions (red are particularly sweet), sliced and separated into rings
Fennel, cut in half lengthways and sliced
Sweet potato, peeled and cut into $\frac{1}{4}$-inch slices
Potatoes, scrubbed and cut into $\frac{1}{4}$-inch slices

Mix together the oil, balsamic vinegar, garlic, oregano, rosemary, salt, and pepper in a bowl until well combined.

Cook the vegetables of your choice on a hot grill for 10 minutes, turning and brushing regularly with the marinade. Serve immediately.

SERVING IDEAS: Serve a selection of grilled vegetables with grilled fish, chicken, or seafood and crusty bread (like baguette or ciabatta, or make bruschetta) accompanied by spreads like aioli, tapenade, or pesto.

Leftover grilled vegetables make a delicious pizza topping or frittata filling, or they can be served as part of an antipasto platter.

Burgers and Hot Dogs

Tuna Burgers

The firm "meaty" texture of tuna makes it ideal to turn into burger patties. In this burger recipe, tuna patties are combined with shredded lettuce, sliced tomatoes, and a Dijon-infused mayonnaise.

SERVES 4

1 scallion (white and green parts), trimmed and roughly chopped
1 tablespoon fresh flat-leaf parsley, chopped
2 tablespoons soy sauce
1 tablespoon extra-virgin olive oil
1 tablespoon freshly squeezed lemon juice
¼ teaspoon ground black pepper
14 ounces (420 g) fresh tuna steaks
2 tablespoons canola oil
4 hamburger buns (regular or whole grain), split open
4 tablespoons Dijon Mayonnaise (page 287)
2 cups shredded iceberg lettuce
2 ripe tomatoes, sliced

Mix together the scallion, parsley, soy sauce, olive oil, lemon juice, and pepper in a small bowl. Cut the tuna into cubes and place in a food processor. Pulse the tuna to break it up. Add the sauce mixture and process until well blended. Form the mixture into 4 patties.

Heat the canola oil in a large skillet over medium heat and cook the patties for 3 minutes on each side. Spread equal amounts of the Dijon Mayonnaise on the bottom of each bun. Top with the lettuce, tomatoes, and a tuna patty. Serve immediately.

Soy Burgers

These meatless burger patties are made with TVP (textured vegetable protein), a healthy nonmeat protein source made from soybeans that's easily prepared and looks and tastes like ground beef.

SERVES 4

¾ cup dried TVP (textured vegetable protein)
¾ cup boiling water
1 large egg, lightly beaten
¼ cup rolled oats (not quick-cooking)
3 tablespoons self-rising flour
¼ onion, finely chopped
1 tablespoon soy sauce
1 tablespoon ketchup
1 teaspoon salt
½ teaspoon ground black pepper
2 tablespoons canola oil
4 tablespoons mayonnaise
4 hamburger buns (regular or whole grain), split open
2 cups shredded iceberg lettuce
2 ripe tomatoes, sliced
2 ounces (60 g) thinly sliced sharp cheddar cheese
12 pickle slices
4 tablespoons ketchup

Pour boiling water over the TVP in a bowl, cover, and set aside for 15 minutes to soak. Mix together the soaked TVP with the egg, oats, flour, onion, soy sauce, ketchup, salt, and pepper until well combined. Shape the mixture into 4 thin, flat patties with wet hands to help prevent sticking.

Heat the oil in a large skillet over medium heat and cook the patties for 3 minutes on each side. Spread equal amounts of the mayonnaise on the bottom of each bun. Top with lettuce, tomatoes, a cooked soy patty, cheese, and pickles. Spread a tablespoon of ketchup on top of each and cover with the bun tops. Serve immediately.

Fish Burgers with Roasted Red Pepper and Wasabi Mayonnaise

The seared fish in these appetizing burgers is enhanced by the sweetness of roasted red pepper and the distinctive bite of wasabi.

SERVES 4

2 tablespoons canola oil
Four 6-ounce (180 g) uncooked firm whitefish fillets (such as snapper, cod, or haddock)
4 tablespoons Wasabi Mayonnaise (page 287)
4 hamburger buns (regular or whole grain), split open
2 cups mixed salad leaves, washed and shaken dry
12 strips of jarred marinated roasted red peppers

Heat the oil in a large skillet over medium heat and cook the fish fillets for 3 minutes on each side. Cut each fillet in half widthways to fit on the bun.

Spread equal amounts of the Wasabi Mayonnaise on the bottom of each bun. Top with the mixed salad leaves, roasted red peppers, and a halved fish fillet and cover with the bun tops. Serve immediately.

VARIATION: Use other fish such as tuna, swordfish, or salmon in place of whitefish fillets, or try chicken breast fillets instead.

Chicken Fillet Burgers with Pesto Mayonnaise

The combination of pesto and mayonnaise makes a luscious dressing that complements seared chicken perfectly.

SERVES 4

2 tablespoons canola oil
Four 6-ounce (180 g) uncooked skinless chicken breast fillets
4 tablespoons Pesto Mayonnaise (page 287)
4 hamburger buns (regular or whole grain), split open

2 cups shredded iceberg lettuce
2 ripe tomatoes, sliced

Heat the oil in a large skillet over medium heat and cook the chicken fillets for 4 minutes each side.

Spread equal amounts of the Pesto Mayonnaise on the bottom of each bun. Top with the lettuce, tomatoes, and a chicken fillet and cover with the bun tops. Serve immediately.

VARIATION: The Pesto Mayonnaise also goes well with fish like swordfish, tuna, or salmon.

▶ Salmon Burgers with Lime Mayonnaise

Pan-fried salmon fillets are combined with arugula leaves, sliced cucumber, and a lime-infused mayonnaise, then encased in fresh soft hamburger buns.

SERVES 4

2 tablespoons canola oil
Four 6-ounce (180 g) fresh salmon fillets
4 tablespoons Lime Mayonnaise (page 287)
4 hamburger buns (regular or whole grain), split open
2 cups loosely packed arugula (rocket), stems trimmed and leaves washed
16 thin cucumber slices

Heat the oil in a large skillet over medium heat and cook the salmon fillets for 3 minutes each side.

Spread equal amounts of the Lime Mayonnaise on the bottom of each bun. Top with the arugula, cucumber, and a salmon fillet and cover with the bun tops. Serve immediately.

Caesar-Style Chicken Fillet Burgers

These burgers combine all the elements of a classic Caesar salad with tender fillets of chicken.

SERVES 4

2 tablespoons canola oil
Four 6-ounce (180 g) uncooked skinless chicken breast fillets
4 lean bacon slices (or soy bacon)
6 tablespoons Caesar Dressing, store-bought
4 hamburger buns (regular or whole grain), split open
2 cups shredded romaine lettuce
2 ripe tomatoes, sliced

Heat the oil in a large skillet over medium heat and cook the chicken fillets for 4 minutes on one side. Turn the chicken over, add the bacon, and cook for another 4 minutes, turning the bacon slices once. Cut each bacon slice in half.

Spread 1½ tablespoons of dressing on the bottom of each bun. Top with the lettuce, tomatoes, a chicken fillet, and bacon and cover with the bun tops. Serve immediately.

Italian-Style Hot Dogs

These are like a cross between hot dogs and pizzas. Soy frankfurters are nestled in buns, spread with an Italian-style tomato sauce; topped with a mixture of cooked onions, peppers, garlic, and mushrooms; and sprinkled with olives and cheese.

SERVES 4

2 tablespoons extra-virgin olive oil
1 onion, finely chopped
1/2 red bell pepper, diced
1/2 green bell pepper, diced
8 white button mushrooms, sliced
2 cloves garlic, finely chopped
4 soy frankfurters
4 hot dog buns (regular or whole grain)
4 tablespoons canned diced tomatoes
2 teaspoons tomato paste
1/2 teaspoon dried oregano
8 pitted black olives, sliced
8 tablespoons grated sharp cheddar cheese

Heat the oil in a skillet over medium heat and cook the onions and bell peppers, stirring occasionally, until softened, about 6 minutes. Add the mushrooms and garlic and cook, stirring occasionally, for another 4 minutes.

Meanwhile, heat the frankfurters according to the package instructions.

Cut a slit down the middle of each hot dog bun and place a frankfurter in each. In a bowl, mix together the canned tomatoes, tomato paste, and oregano. Top each hot dog with the tomato sauce, then top with the cooked vegetables, olives, and cheese. Serve immediately.

Chili Hot Dogs

A spicy version of a Western favorite—topped with cooked onions, red pepper, salsa, and cheese.

SERVES 4

2 tablespoons canola oil
1 onion, finely chopped
1 red bell pepper, diced
4 soy frankfurters
4 hot dog buns (regular or whole grain)
4 tablespoons Mexican salsa
8 tablespoons grated sharp cheddar cheese

Heat the oil in a skillet over medium heat and cook the onion and bell pepper, stirring occasionally, until softened, about 6 minutes.

Meanwhile, heat the frankfurters according to the package instructions.

Cut a slit down the middle of each hot dog bun and place a frankfurter in each. Top each hot dog with salsa, then top with the cooked onions and peppers and some cheese. Serve immediately.

Sandwiches and Wraps

Italian-Style Chicken Sandwich with Pesto Mayonnaise

Italian breads, like focaccia and ciabatta, are popular alternatives to ordinary sliced bread. In this sandwich, the bread is split, spread with pesto-flavored mayonnaise, and filled with roast chicken, arugula, sun-dried tomatoes, and olives.

SERVES 4

4 tablespoons mayonnaise
2 tablespoons pesto, homemade (page 278) or store-bought
1 Italian-style bread loaf such as ciabatta or focaccia, cut in half lengthways
2 cups loosely packed arugula (rocket), stems trimmed and leaves washed
12 ounces (360 g) shredded roast chicken breast
8 sun-dried tomatoes, sliced
8 pitted black olives, sliced

Mix together the mayonnaise and the pesto in a small bowl. Spread the pesto-mayonnaise mixture over the base of the ciabatta or focaccia loaf. Top with the arugula leaves, chicken, sun-dried tomatoes, and black olives. Cover with the top half of the loaf and cut into quarters to serve.

VARIATION: Replace the arugula with mixed salad leaves, and use strips of roasted red pepper instead of sun-dried tomatoes.

Focaccia with Smoked Salmon and Avocado

Focaccia stuffed with tender smoked salmon slices, creamy avocado, and crisp salad vegetables.

SERVES 4

7 ounces (200 g) sliced smoked salmon
1 focaccia bread, cut in half lengthways
2 ripe tomatoes, sliced
1 avocado, sliced
12 thinly sliced rings of red onion

2 cups green mignonette or butter lettuce leaves
2 tablespoons freshly squeezed lemon juice
2 tablespoons extra-virgin olive oil
½ clove garlic, minced
½ teaspoon sea salt
½ teaspoon freshly ground black pepper

Arrange equal amounts of the smoked salmon on the base of the focaccia. Top with the tomato, avocado, red onions, and lettuce. In a small bowl, mix together the lemon juice, oil, garlic, salt, and pepper. Drizzle the dressing over the top, cover with the top half of the focaccia, and cut into quarters to serve.

▶ Hummus and Salad Wraps

Hummus is a healthy alternative to butter or margarine and combines perfectly with flat bread, salad, and cheese to make this tasty wrap.

SERVES 4

4 heaping tablespoons hummus, homemade (page 284) or store-bought
4 whole grain flat breads (such as lavash, pocketless pita bread, or tortilla)
½ cup grated sharp cheddar cheese
2 cups shredded iceberg lettuce
2 small carrots, peeled and grated
2 ripe tomatoes, chopped
2 scallions (white and green parts), trimmed and thinly sliced
Sea salt and freshly ground black pepper to taste

Spread equal amounts of hummus in a horizontal line down the middle of each flat bread. Arrange the cheese, lettuce, carrots, tomatoes, and scallions on top of the hummus. Season with salt and pepper, roll up, and cut each wrap in half to serve.

VARIATION: Wrap other salad vegetables in the hummus-spread flat breads— onion, radish, red and green bell peppers, avocado, and sprouts (such as alfalfa or snow pea) are all tasty additions.

Greek Salad Pita Pockets

Pita bread is a versatile alternative to standard sliced bread, and it can be cut in half then opened up to form neat pockets, ready to be stuffed with the filling of your choice. In this recipe, pita bread is filled with a combination of traditional Greek salad and velvety smooth hummus to make a delicious and nutritious meal-in-a-pocket.

SERVES 4

2 cups shredded romaine (cos) lettuce
2 ripe tomatoes, finely chopped
1 cup finely diced cucumber
16 thin slices red onion
$\frac{1}{2}$ green bell pepper, finely diced
8 pitted black olives (kalamata are particularly good), sliced
2 ounces (60 g) crumbled feta cheese
1 tablespoon extra-virgin olive oil
1 tablespoon freshly squeezed lemon juice
$\frac{1}{4}$ teaspoon sea salt
$\frac{1}{4}$ teaspoon freshly ground black pepper
8 tablespoons hummus, homemade (page 284) or store-bought
4 whole-grain pita breads, cut in half and opened into pockets

In a bowl, mix together the lettuce, tomatoes, cucumber, onions, bell pepper, olives, cheese, oil, lemon juice, salt, and pepper until well combined. Spread 2 tablespoons of hummus inside each pita and fill with equal amounts of the filling to serve.

Tuna and Sweet Chili Wraps

This healthy sandwich wrap embraces the exotic flavors of Thailand.

SERVES 4

2 tablespoons mayonnaise
2 tablespoons sweet chili sauce
1 tablespoon finely chopped cilantro (fresh coriander)
12 ounces (360 g) canned tuna in vegetable oil, drained and flaked
4 whole-grain flat breads (such as lavash, pocketless pita bread, or tortilla)
2 cups shredded iceberg lettuce

2 carrots, peeled and grated
1 cup finely diced cucumber

Mix together the mayonnaise, sweet chili sauce, and cilantro in a bowl and stir in the tuna. Spread the tuna mixture in a horizontal line down the middle of each flat bread. Arrange equal amounts of lettuce, carrots, and cucumber on top of the tuna mixture. Roll up firmly and cut each in half to serve.

VARIATION: Replace the tuna with 2 cups of shredded skinless cooked chicken breast.

▶ ## Turkish Chickpea Salad Wrap

There are three parts to this easy-to-assemble Middle Eastern wrap: the flat bread, the hummus, and the chickpea salad. The combination of all three makes a healthy and substantial no-cook feast you can hold in your hands.

SERVES 4

2 cups canned chickpeas, rinsed and drained
½ small red onion, finely chopped
1 red bell pepper, diced
2 tablespoons finely chopped cilantro (fresh coriander)
1 teaspoon freshly grated lemon zest
2 tablespoons extra-virgin olive oil
4 whole-grain flat breads (such as lavash, pocketless pita bread, or tortilla)
8 tablespoons hummus, homemade (page 284) or store-bought
2 handfuls torn romaine lettuce

Mix together the chickpeas, onion, bell pepper, cilantro, lemon zest, and oil in a bowl. Spread the hummus in a horizontal line down the middle of each flat bread. Arrange the lettuce over the hummus and top with the chickpea mixture. Roll up firmly and cut each in half to serve.

Bruschetta with Tomato, Mozzarella, and Anchovy

Bruschetta is sliced toasted bread, rubbed with garlic and drizzled or brushed with olive oil. It makes the perfect base for this classic Mediterranean combination of juicy tomatoes, fresh basil, creamy mozzarella, and salty anchovies.

SERVES 4

8 thick slices of crusty bread such as ciabatta or baguette
   (sliced on the diagonal)
1 clove garlic, peeled and cut in half
2 tablespoons extra-virgin olive oil
4 ripe tomatoes, finely diced
6 anchovy fillets, chopped
¼ teaspoon sea salt
¼ teaspoon freshly ground black pepper
4 ounces (120 g) fresh mozzarella cheese, thinly sliced
8 large fresh basil leaves, roughly torn

Preheat the oven broiler (griller).

Toast bread on both sides under the broiler. Rub the surface of each slice with the cut side of the garlic. Brush or drizzle each slice, on one side only, with a little extra-virgin olive oil.

In a bowl, mix together the tomatoes, anchovies, salt, and pepper and place on top of the toasts. Top with cheese, place under the broiler, and cook until the cheese is bubbly and golden. Sprinkle with basil and serve immediately.

Mushroom Bruschetta

Bruschetta topped with panfried mushrooms seasoned with sea salt, freshly ground black pepper, and flat-leaf parsley. This recipe serves four as a light meal or eight as an appetizer.

SERVES 4

3 tablespoons extra-virgin olive oil plus 4 teaspoons for drizzling

4 cups sliced portobello mushrooms

8 thick slices of ciabatta (Italian crusty bread), or use baguette sliced
   on the diagonal instead

1 clove garlic, peeled and cut in half

2 tablespoons finely chopped flat-leaf parsley

1 teaspoon sea salt

$\frac{1}{2}$ teaspoon freshly ground black pepper

Preheat the oven broiler (griller).

Heat 2 tablespoons of the oil in a skillet over medium heat. Add the mushrooms and cook, stirring regularly, until softened, 4 to 5 minutes.

While the mushrooms are cooking, toast the ciabatta slices under the broiler until golden on both sides. Rub one side of each slice of ciabatta with the cut side of garlic. Brush or drizzle each slice, on one side only, with half a teaspoon of oil.

Off the heat, add the reserved tablespoon of oil, the parsley, salt, and pepper to the skillet with the mushrooms and stir. Spoon equal amounts on top of each bruschetta and serve immediately.

Pan Bagnat

Literally meaning "bathed bread," this sandwich, which originates from the Provence region of southern France, makes great picnic fare and can be made up the night before to allow the flavors to mingle.

SERVES 4

6 tablespoons extra-virgin olive oil

2 tablespoons white wine vinegar

1 teaspoon Dijon mustard

1 clove garlic, minced

1 teaspoon salt

$\frac{1}{2}$ teaspoon freshly ground black pepper

1 large baguette

12 ounces (360 g) canned tuna in olive oil, drained and broken into chunks

$\frac{1}{2}$ green bell pepper, diced

2 ripe tomatoes, sliced

3 large eggs, hard-boiled, peeled and sliced

15 half rings of red onion

12 pitted black olives, sliced

Place the oil, vinegar, mustard, garlic, salt, and pepper in a jar with screw-top lid and shake until well combined. Cut the baguette in half lengthways and remove some of the soft bread from the center of each half to hollow out a little. Arrange the tuna, bell pepper, tomatoes, eggs, onions, and olives on the bottom half, then drizzle with the dressing. Top with the other baguette half and wrap tightly with plastic wrap and refrigerate for at least 1 hour to allow the flavors to develop. Bring to room temperature before cutting into quarters to serve.

Soups

Minestrone Soup

This classic Italian minestrone soup is packed with flavor and nutrients and is hearty enough to be eaten as a light meal in its own right.

4 tablespoons extra-virgin olive oil
2 slices lean bacon, finely chopped
1 red onion, diced
1 carrot, peeled and diced
1 stick celery, diced
2 cloves garlic, minced
6 cups vegetable stock
2 cups chopped canned whole tomatoes
1 teaspoon sea salt
½ teaspoon freshly ground black pepper
½ cup small pasta, such as elbows or orzo
½ cup frozen green peas, thawed
1 zucchini (courgette), cut in half lengthways and thinly sliced into half-moons
1 cup canned white beans (like cannellini), rinsed and drained
2 tablespoons finely chopped fresh parsley
Finely grated Parmesan or Romano cheese

Heat 2 tablespoons of the oil in a large saucepan and cook the bacon, stirring occasionally, for 2 minutes. Add the onion, carrot, and celery and cook, covered, for 3 minutes. Stir again and cook, covered, for another 3 minutes. Add the garlic and cook, stirring regularly, for a minute. Add the stock, tomatoes, salt, and pepper and stir to combine. Bring to a boil, cover, reduce the heat to medium, and simmer for 10 minutes.

Add the pasta, peas, zucchini, and beans, stir to combine; increase the heat to medium–high and cook, covered, until pasta is tender, about 10 minutes. Remove from the heat and stir in the parsley and the reserved 2 tablespoons of olive oil. Serve in bowls sprinkled with a little grated Parmesan or Romano cheese.

TIP: If you don't eat meat, use soy bacon in place of real bacon.

Tuscan White Bean and Garlic Soup

The garlic used in this recipe becomes surprisingly sweet and soft as it cooks and makes this heart-warming soup extra heart-healthy.

SERVES 4

6 tablespoons extra-virgin olive oil

2 onions, chopped

28 ounces (840 g) canned white beans (like cannellini), rinsed and drained

2 potatoes, peeled and cut into bite-size cubes

8 cloves unpeeled garlic

1 teaspoon dried rosemary

10 cups chicken or vegetable stock

2 teaspoons sea salt

1 teaspoon freshly ground black pepper

Heat 4 tablespoons of the olive oil in a large saucepan over medium heat. Add the onions and cook, stirring, until softened, about 6 minutes. Add the beans, potatoes, garlic, and rosemary and cook for a minute, stirring to combine. Add the stock, salt, and pepper, bring to a boil, and cover with a lid. Reduce the heat to medium-low and simmer gently for 20 minutes, stirring once or twice.

Remove the garlic cloves and rinse them briefly under cold water. Squeeze the soft cooked garlic from each clove into a blender or food processor. Pour in half the soup and blend for about 15 seconds until smooth. Return the puree to the soup, stir in the reserved oil, and heat through before serving.

Miso Soup with Tofu and Mushroom

This nourishing Japanese soup takes only minutes to prepare and can be served for breakfast, lunch, or as part of a main meal. Miso—fermented soy bean paste—adds a rich flavor and is highly valued in Japan for its health-giving properties.

SERVES 4

6 cups dashi stock (dashi stock powder is available at Asian food stores)
4 thinly sliced fresh mushrooms (shiitake or white button)
3 tablespoons red or white miso paste
2 tablespoons Japanese soy sauce
3 ounces (90 g) silken tofu, cut into cubes
1 scallion (white and green parts), trimmed and thinly sliced on the diagonal

Bring the stock to a gentle boil in a saucepan, add the mushrooms, reduce the heat and simmer for 3 minutes.

Mix together the miso and soy sauce in a small bowl, then add to the hot stock. Add the tofu. Heat the soup and, just before it comes to a boil, remove from the heat. Pour the soup into bowls and garnish with the sliced scallions on top to serve.

VARIATION: You can add various other ingredients to make a more substantial soup, such as cooked shrimp, snow pea sprouts, cooked rice noodles, or paper-thin slices of fresh ginger.

Soupe au Pistou

A thick, rich Provençal vegetable and bean soup infused with fresh basil. This soup is a meal in itself served with crusty bread.

SERVES 4

2 tablespoons extra-virgin olive oil
1 onion, cut in half, thinly sliced, and separated into half-rings
1 carrot, peeled, quartered lengthways, and thinly sliced
1 zucchini (courgette), halved lengthways and sliced into ½-inch rounds
1 potato, peeled and cut into bite-size pieces
1 cup green beans, ends trimmed, cut into 1-inch pieces
6 cups chicken or vegetable stock
½ teaspoon sea salt
¼ teaspoon freshly ground black pepper
14 ounces (420 g) canned white beans (like cannellini), rinsed and drained
3 tablespoons pesto, store-bought or homemade

Heat the oil in a large saucepan over a medium heat. Add the onion and carrot and cook, stirring, for 3 minutes. Add the zucchini, potato, and green beans and cook, stirring occasionally, for another 2 minutes. Add the stock, salt, and pepper, bring to a boil, then cover the pot, reduce the heat, and simmer for 15 minutes. Add the white beans and pesto and cook for 5 minutes. Serve in bowls with crusty bread on the side.

Gazpacho

There are about as many gazpacho recipes as there are Spanish cooks. This is our quick version, which requires little effort but produces an authentic result. This cold soup is delicious and refreshing—a perfect summertime meal served with bread.

SERVES 4

6 cups tomato juice
2 cups peeled, deseeded and chopped cucumber
1 small red onion, chopped
1 red bell pepper, deseeded and chopped
1 green bell pepper, deseeded and chopped
1 clove garlic, chopped
2 tablespoons extra-virgin olive oil
2 teaspoons white wine vinegar
1 teaspoon sea salt
½ teaspoon ground black pepper

Place all ingredients in a food processor or blender and process until smooth. Chill in the fridge until you're ready to serve.

VARIATIONS: If you like a spicy kick, add a few drops of Tabasco sauce.

You can use ripe and flavorful fresh tomatoes instead of tomato juice, but you need to skin and deseed them first (which is why we prefer to use good-quality tomato juice).

TIP: The flavors of gazpacho develop over time, so allow the soup to chill in the fridge for at least 20 minutes, and up to a day ahead of time.

▶ Pho Bo

Pho bo is a Vietnamese beef and noodle soup that is often eaten for breakfast but also makes a satisfying lunch or light dinner. The boiling stock, fragrant with spices and sauces, is poured over the noodles, bean sprouts, and scallions, and it poaches the paper-thin slices of raw beef just before serving.

SERVES 4

4 ounces (120 g) dried rice stick noodles
8 cups beef stock
1 onion, finely chopped
4 tablespoons hoisin sauce
2 tablespoons fish sauce
2 teaspoons finely grated fresh ginger
1 teaspoon ground black pepper
1 teaspoon five-spice powder
2 cups bean sprouts
2 scallions (white and green parts), trimmed and thinly sliced
10 ounces (300 g) very thinly sliced bite-size lean beef
2 tablespoons freshly squeezed lemon juice
Cilantro (fresh coriander) leaves, for garnish
Strips of fresh red chile, for garnish

Soak the noodles in a bowl of boiling water for 10 minutes.

Place the stock, onion, hoisin sauce, fish sauce, ginger, pepper, and five-spice powder in a saucepan. Bring to a boil, cover, and simmer over a medium heat for 10 minutes.

Drain the noodles and place equal amounts into soup bowls. Place equal amounts of the sprouts, scallions, and beef slices on top of the noodles. Pour over the boiling stock to cover and allow to stand for 1 minute to poach, ensuring the beef is immersed. Serve the soup drizzled with lemon juice and garnished with cilantro leaves and chile strips on top.

VARIATION: Use thinly sliced firm tofu or smoked salmon instead of beef.

TIP: To help cut the beef into paper-thin slices, place the meat in the freezer for about 30 minutes to firm up before slicing with a very sharp knife.

Greek Spinach and White Bean Soup

A delicately seasoned Greek soup with white beans and a range of vegetables including spinach, carrots, onion, celery, and potato. This soup can be served as an appetizer, or enjoyed as a light meal with crusty bread for dipping.

SERVES 4

3 tablespoons extra-virgin olive oil
1 onion, diced
1 carrot, peeled and diced
1 stick celery, diced
1 potato, peeled and diced
1 clove garlic, finely chopped
6 cups vegetable stock
2 tablespoons finely chopped fresh flat-leaf parsley
14 ounces (420 g) canned white beans (like cannellini), rinsed and drained
8 ounces (240 g) package frozen spinach, defrosted and drained
$\frac{1}{2}$ cup frozen green peas, thawed
1 teaspoon salt
$\frac{1}{2}$ teaspoon freshly ground black pepper

Heat 2 tablespoons of the oil in a large saucepan and cook the onion, carrot, and celery, stirring occasionally, until softened, about 5 minutes. Add the potato and garlic and cook, stirring, for 1 minute. Add the stock and parsley, bring to a boil, then reduce the heat to medium and simmer for 15 minutes. Add the white beans, spinach, peas, salt, and pepper, return to a simmer, and cook for another 5 minutes. Remove from the heat, stir in the remaining tablespoon of oil, and serve.

Spanish Broccoli and Almond Soup

The combination of ground almonds and broccoli makes a deliciously creamy yet creamless soup with a rich, green color.

10 cups vegetable stock
8 cups broccoli florets
2 red onions, roughly chopped
2 medium-sized potatoes, peeled and cut into small cubes
1 cup ground almonds
2 cloves garlic, roughly chopped
2 teaspoons sea salt
1 teaspoon freshly ground black pepper
2 tablespoons extra-virgin olive oil

Place the stock, broccoli, onions, potatoes, almonds, garlic, salt, and pepper in a large saucepan and bring to a boil. Cover the pot, reduce the heat to medium, and simmer for 15 minutes. Transfer the soup to a blender and process until smooth, then return to the saucepan. Stir in the olive oil and heat thoroughly before serving.

SERVING IDEA: You can also chill this soup and serve it cold as a light summer meal with bread.

Tunisian Chickpea and Vegetable Soup

This hearty chickpea and vegetable soup is flavored with warm spices including saffron, cumin, cinnamon, ground ginger, and turmeric. The addition of cilantro, parsley, and lemon juice toward the end of cooking adds a fresh herb-citrus taste, while the pasta adds body and texture.

SERVES 4

2 tablespoons extra-virgin olive oil
1 onion, finely chopped
1 stick celery, finely chopped
1 teaspoon salt
$\frac{1}{2}$ teaspoon turmeric
$\frac{1}{2}$ teaspoon ground ginger
$\frac{1}{2}$ teaspoon cinnamon
$\frac{1}{2}$ teaspoon ground cumin
$\frac{1}{2}$ teaspoon ground black pepper
1 zucchini (courgette), sliced into thin rounds
14 ounces (420 g) canned whole tomatoes, chopped
$\frac{1}{2}$ cup red lentils
$5\frac{1}{2}$ cups vegetable stock
$\frac{1}{4}$ teaspoon saffron strands, soaked in $\frac{1}{2}$ cup boiling water
1 cup canned chickpeas, rinsed and drained
1 ounce capellini (angel-hair) pasta, broken into pieces
2 tablespoons chopped cilantro (fresh coriander)
2 tablespoons chopped fresh flat-leaf parsley
2 tablespoons freshly squeezed lemon juice

Heat the oil in a large saucepan over a medium heat. Add the onion and celery and cook, stirring occasionally, until softened, about 5 minutes. Add the salt, turmeric, ginger, cinnamon, cumin, and pepper and cook, stirring, for 1 minute. Add the zucchini, tomatoes, and lentils and stir to combine. Add the stock and saffron liquid and bring to a boil. Cover the pot, reduce the heat to medium, and simmer for 15 minutes.

Add the chickpeas, pasta, cilantro, parsley, and lemon juice and stir to combine. Cook, covered, for 5 minutes and serve.

Thai-Spiced Sweet Potato Soup

A velvety-smooth soup accented with Thai seasonings. The sweet potato adds not only texture and a vivid color to the soup but also a healthy dose of beta-carotene and dietary fiber.

SERVES 4

1 tablespoon canola or peanut oil
1 onion, chopped
3 cloves garlic, chopped
2 teaspoons red curry paste
5 cups chicken or vegetable stock
1 cup coconut milk
3 tablespoons fish sauce
2 pounds orange sweet potatoes, peeled and roughly chopped
1 cup red lentils
2 teaspoons brown sugar
2 tablespoons freshly squeezed lemon juice
Cilantro (fresh coriander) leaves, for garnish

Heat the oil in a large saucepan over a medium heat. Add the onion and cook, stirring occasionally, until softened, about 5 minutes. Add the garlic and red curry paste and cook, stirring constantly, for 1 minute. Add the stock, coconut milk, fish sauce, sweet potatoes, red lentils, and brown sugar, stir to combine, and bring to a boil. Reduce the heat to medium and simmer, covered, for 20 minutes. Remove from the heat and allow to cool a little. Puree the soup in two batches in a blender or food processor until smooth. Return to the saucepan to reheat and stir in the lemon juice. Serve in bowls garnished with cilantro.

VARIATIONS: Replace the sweet potatoes with butternut squash (or pumpkin).

Substitute lime juice for the lemon juice.

Use yellow split peas rather than red lentils (in which case you'll need to cook for about 35 minutes).

Southeast Asian Hot and Sour Shrimp Soup

This spicy shrimp soup is quick and easy to prepare and can be served as a nutritious meal in itself.

SERVES 4

4 teaspoons canola or peanut oil
2 teaspoons Thai red curry paste
2 teaspoons finely chopped lemongrass or lemon zest
1 clove garlic, finely chopped
1 cup sliced mushrooms
8 cups chicken stock
16 uncooked shrimp (prawns), peeled (bottom part of tails left on
    if desired) and deveined
4 ounces (120 g) rice vermicelli noodles
2 tablespoons fish sauce
3 tablespoons freshly squeezed lemon juice
2 teaspoons brown sugar
2 scallions (white and green parts), trimmed and thinly sliced
2 tablespoons finely chopped cilantro (fresh coriander)
2 small red chiles, sliced into thin rounds

Heat the oil in a large saucepan over a medium heat. Add the curry paste, lemongrass or zest, and garlic and cook, stirring, for 30 seconds. Add the mushrooms and cook for 1 minute, then add the stock and bring to a boil. Add the shrimp and noodles and simmer for 3 minutes. Add the fish sauce, lemon juice, and sugar, and simmer gently for another minute. Stir in the scallions and cilantro just before serving, and garnish with the sliced chiles.

VARIATION: Use cubed tofu or bite-size pieces of skinless chicken breast fillets in place of the shrimp.

Salads

Japanese Soba Noodle Salad

Soba noodles combined with creamy avocado, a selection of crisp vegetables, and a Japanese soy-ginger dressing.

5 ounces (150 g) dried soba noodles
5 tablespoons Japanese soy sauce
3 tablespoons Japanese rice vinegar
1½ tablespoons finely grated fresh ginger
1 teaspoon sugar
20 thinly sliced rounds of cucumber, cut into halves
15 snow peas, ends trimmed and cut in half on the diagonal
1 carrot, peeled and grated
1 scallion (white and green parts), trimmed and thinly sliced on the diagonal
1 avocado, peeled and cut into small cubes

Cook the noodles in boiling water for 4 minutes, rinse under cold water, drain, and set aside.

Mix together the soy sauce, rice vinegar, ginger, and sugar in a small bowl. Place the noodles in the bottom of a large mixing bowl. Add the cucumber, snow peas, carrot, scallion, and avocado. Drizzle with the soy dressing, toss gently to combine, and serve.

VARIATIONS: Add strips of smoked salmon to this salad for a more opulent version.

For added bite, mix 1 teaspoon of wasabi into the dressing.

Greek Salad

Greek salad, or *horiatiki*, is a rough country salad of juicy tomatoes, crisp cucumber, sliced red onion, green bell pepper, crumbly feta cheese, and plump kalamata olives. Serve this delightful combination as a side dish or as a light meal with some crusty bread.

SERVES 4

3 tablespoons extra-virgin olive oil
1½ tablespoons freshly squeezed lemon juice
1 clove garlic, minced
½ teaspoon dried oregano
¼ teaspoon sea salt
¼ teaspoon freshly ground black pepper, and extra for garnish
3 ripe tomatoes, cut into wedges
¼ red onion, sliced into rings
½ cucumber, sliced lengthwise, then cut into thick half-moons
½ green bell pepper, julienned
16 pitted kalamata olives
4 ounces (120 g) feta cheese, cut into small cubes

Place the olive oil, lemon juice, garlic, oregano, salt, and pepper in a small jar with a screw-top lid and shake to combine.

Place the tomatoes, onion, cucumber, bell pepper, olives, and cheese in a large bowl. Pour the dressing over the salad and toss gently to combine, just before serving. Garnish with a little freshly ground black pepper.

Salade Niçoise

This classic Provençal salad explodes with flavor and is also a powerhouse of valuable nutrients: the tuna and anchovies provide protein and are a rich source of omega-3 fatty acids, the olives and olive oil supply heart-healthy monounsaturated fat, the eggs provide protein and vitamins, the potatoes provide energy-giving carbohydrates, as well as plenty of potassium and fiber, and the salad vegetables add more fiber as well as a healthy dose of phytochemicals and antioxidants. Talk about good food that's good for you!

SERVES 4

2 small potatoes, peeled and cut into bite-size cubes
16 green beans, ends trimmed and halved
4 cups butter lettuce leaves, washed and dried
14 ounces (420 g) canned light meat tuna in olive oil, drained and broken into chunks
2 ripe tomatoes, cut into wedges
¼ red onion, thinly sliced and separated into rings
3 large eggs, hard-boiled, peeled and quartered
16 pitted black olives (Niçoise are ideal)
4 anchovy fillets, halved lengthways
3 tablespoons extra-virgin olive oil
2 tablespoons red or white wine vinegar
1 clove garlic, minced
½ teaspoon Dijon mustard
½ teaspoon salt
½ teaspoon freshly ground black pepper

In a steamer basket over simmering water, steam the potatoes until tender, 8 to 10 minutes, adding the beans for the last 5 minutes of cooking, then set aside to cool.

Arrange the lettuce, potatoes, beans, tuna, tomatoes, onion, eggs, olives, and anchovies on a serving platter.

Place the oil, vinegar, garlic, mustard, salt, and pepper in a small jar with a screw-top lid and shake to combine. Pour the dressing evenly over the salad to serve.

VARIATION: For a more opulent version, you can poach or grill fresh fillets of salmon or tuna, allow to cool, and cut into cubes to replace the canned tuna.

▶ Insalata di Riso (Italian Rice Salad)

A hearty Italian rice salad packed with tasty and healthful ingredients including tuna, tomatoes, toasted pine nuts, mushrooms, peas, cubed mozzarella cheese, artichoke hearts, and diced green bell pepper. This salad can be served as a side dish or eaten in larger quantities as a light meal.

SERVES 4

1 cup long-grain white rice, cooked and left to cool (or use leftover rice)
2 artichoke hearts (jarred or canned), roughly chopped
6 ounces (180 g) canned light meat tuna in olive oil, drained and broken into chunks
$\frac{1}{3}$ cup frozen peas, cooked and cooled
1 large ripe tomato, diced
$\frac{1}{4}$ cup cubed mozzarella cheese
$\frac{1}{4}$ green bell pepper, diced
2 white button mushrooms, thinly sliced
2 tablespoons pine nuts, lightly toasted
2 tablespoons finely chopped fresh flat-leaf parsley
4 tablespoons extra-virgin olive oil
$1\frac{1}{2}$ tablespoons freshly squeezed lemon juice
1 clove garlic, finely chopped
1 teaspoon salt
$\frac{1}{2}$ teaspoon freshly ground black pepper

Mix together the rice, artichoke hearts, tuna, peas, tomato, cheese, bell pepper, mushrooms, pine nuts, and parsley in a bowl.

Mix together the oil, lemon juice, garlic, salt, and pepper in a small bowl until well combined (or shake together in a screw-top jar). Pour the dressing over the rice mixture, mix together gently to combine thoroughly, and serve.

VARIATION: You can vary this salad endlessly—add black or green olives, sun-dried tomatoes, capers, or use red bell peppers instead of green or finely chopped basil instead of parsley.

Pesto Pasta Salad with White Beans, Cherry Tomatoes, and Artichoke Hearts

Traditional pesto Genoese made with basil and pine nuts is ideal for this tasty pasta salad.

SERVES 4

8 ounces (240 g) pasta of your choice (shells or spirals are ideal)
¾ cup of pesto, homemade (page 278) or store-bought
8 ounces (240 g) cherry tomatoes, cut in half
1 cup canned cannellini beans, rinsed and drained
1 cup jarred quartered artichoke hearts

Cook the pasta in a large pot of boiling water, according to package directions. Drain the cooked pasta, and refresh under cold water. Toss the pasta with the pesto, cherry tomatoes, cannellini beans, and artichoke hearts until well combined.

VARIATION: Replace the cannellini beans with 1 cup of shredded cooked chicken breast and add some sliced black olives.

Turkish Tomato, Cucumber, and Olive Salad

A simple combination of fresh tomatoes, cucumber, and black olives tossed with a tangy dressing made with lemon juice, vinegar, and olive oil.

SERVES 4

4 tablespoons extra-virgin olive oil
4 teaspoons freshly squeezed lemon juice
2 teaspoons white wine vinegar
2 teaspoons finely chopped fresh flat-leaf parsley
¼ teaspoon sea salt
¼ teaspoon freshly ground black pepper
4 ripe tomatoes, sliced
24 thinly sliced rounds of cucumber
12 pitted black olives, sliced

Mix together the oil, lemon juice, vinegar, parsley, salt, and pepper in a bowl until well combined.

Place the tomatoes, cucumber, and olives in a salad bowl. Pour the dressing over the salad and toss gently to combine just before serving.

▶ Tabbouleh

A traditional Middle Eastern salad made with chopped fresh herbs (mainly flat-leaf parsley but also mint), bulgur, diced tomato, and scallion and dressed with extra-virgin olive oil and lemon juice. This recipe involves a lot of chopping, but the herbs can also be chopped using a food processor—just be sure to use the pulse button with discretion, or the herbs will start to turn into a paste.

SERVES 4

½ cup bulgur
1½ cups finely chopped flat-leaf parsley
2 ripe tomatoes, diced
1½ tablespoons finely chopped fresh mint
2 scallions (white and green parts), trimmed and finely sliced
¼ cup extra-virgin olive oil
3 tablespoons freshly squeezed lemon juice
1 teaspoon salt
¼ teaspoon ground black pepper

Mix the bulgur with ¾ cup of water in a saucepan. Bring to a boil, cover, then turn the heat on very low and cook for 15 minutes. Fluff with a fork to separate the grains, then allow to cool while preparing the other ingredients.

Place the bulgur in a salad bowl with the parsley, tomatoes, mint, scallions, oil, lemon juice, salt, and pepper. Toss well to combine and serve.

Panzanella (Tuscan Bread Salad)

This classic Tuscan summer dish uses day-old bread that is torn into pieces, softened with water, then mixed with tomatoes, fresh basil, red onion, and a simple olive oil vinaigrette.

SERVES 4

4 cups cubed day-old Italian ciabatta bread
4 ripe tomatoes, diced
4 tablespoons finely chopped red onion
16 basil leaves, roughly torn
6 tablespoons extra-virgin olive oil
4 tablespoons red wine vinegar
1 clove garlic, minced
1 teaspoon sea salt
½ teaspoon freshly ground black pepper

Place the bread in a bowl, cover with water, and soak for 5 minutes until softened. Remove handfuls of the bread at a time and squeeze dry. Place the bread in a bowl with the tomatoes, red onion, and basil.

Mix together the oil, vinegar, garlic, salt, and pepper in a small bowl until well combined. Pour the dressing over the salad, toss gently to combine, and serve.

Gado Gado

Gado gado is an Indonesian salad made with green beans, potatoes, carrots, cabbage, and bean sprouts garnished with sliced boiled eggs and drizzled with a luscious peanut sauce. Gado gado is such a hearty and filling salad that it can easily be eaten as a complete meal.

SERVES 4

2 cups Indonesian Peanut Sauce (page 282)
2 potatoes, peeled and cubed
2 carrots, peeled and julienned
20 green beans, ends trimmed
¼ head cauliflower, broken into small florets
2 cups shredded cabbage
2 cups bean sprouts
4 large eggs, hard-boiled, shelled, and cut into quarters

While the peanut sauce is simmering, bring a large saucepan of lightly salted water to a boil. Add the potatoes and cook for 3 minutes. Add the carrots, green beans, and cauliflower and boil for another 4 minutes. Add the cabbage and bean sprouts and boil for 2 minutes. Drain the vegetables and rinse under cold water to refresh.

Arrange equal amounts of each vegetable on plates, garnish with egg quarters, and drizzle with peanut sauce to serve.

TIP: Allow the water to return to a rolling boil after adding each vegetable to ensure they are cooked according to the times allocated.

Thai Chicken Salad

Strips of chicken breast and a selection of colorful vegetables served with a lemon juice and sweet chile dressing.

SERVES 4

8 handfuls of green mignonette or butter lettuce, washed and dried

28 thinly sliced rounds of peeled cucumber

½ red bell pepper, very thinly julienned

1 carrot, peeled and grated

12 ounces (360 g) precooked chicken breast, skin removed and flesh
   torn into strips

4 tablespoons fish sauce

2 tablespoons sweet chili sauce

2 tablespoons freshly squeezed lemon juice

2 teaspoons sesame oil

1 clove garlic, minced

2 tablespoons finely chopped fresh mint

Arrange the lettuce, cucumber, bell pepper, carrot, and chicken on a serving platter.

Mix together the fish sauce, chili sauce, lemon juice, sesame oil, and garlic in a small bowl until well combined. Drizzle the dressing over the salad and garnish with mint to serve.

Breakfasts

Tuna, Pea, and Corn Frittata

Frittata is the Italian equivalent of an omelet. This specialty is very easy to prepare and is ideal either as a hearty breakfast served with slices of lightly buttered whole grain toast or plain bruschetta or eaten as a delightful light dinner with a salad and some crusty bread.

SERVES 2

1 1/2 tablespoons extra-virgin olive oil
1/2 onion, finely chopped
1/4 cup frozen green peas, thawed
1/4 cup corn kernels
1/2 clove garlic, minced
3 ounces (90 g) canned tuna in olive oil, drained and flaked
4 large eggs
1/2 tablespoon chopped fresh flat-leaf parsley
1/2 teaspoon sea salt
1/4 teaspoon freshly ground black pepper
1/4 cup grated Parmesan cheese

Preheat the oven broiler (griller).

Heat 1 tablespoon of the oil in a medium-size skillet over medium heat and cook the onion, stirring occasionally, for 3 minutes. Add the peas, corn, and garlic and cook, stirring occasionally, for another 3 minutes. Transfer the mixture to a bowl, mix in the flaked tuna, and allow to cool slightly.

Whisk the eggs in a bowl with the parsley, salt, and pepper, then mix together with the tuna and vegetable mixture.

Heat the remaining oil in the skillet over medium heat, then pour in the egg, tuna, and vegetable mixture. Cook the frittata gently over a low heat, covered, about 8 minutes. Sprinkle the top with the cheese and cook under the preheated broiler for 1 minute. Cut the frittata into wedges and serve.

VARIATIONS: Prepare the frittata with 2 thin slices of diced ham in place of the tuna.

Try other vegetables like zucchini (courgette) or red and green bell peppers.

Tortilla de Patatas

Tortilla is a traditional Spanish egg dish similar to a French omelet and an Italian frittata. This version includes potatoes, red onion, and green bell peppers.

SERVES 2

1 potato, peeled and cut into small cubes
2 tablespoons extra-virgin olive oil
½ red onion, finely chopped
½ green bell pepper, deseeded and finely diced
4 large eggs
1 tablespoon finely chopped fresh flat-leaf parsley
½ teaspoon sea salt
¼ teaspoon freshly ground black pepper

Preheat the oven broiler (griller).

Steam the potato in a steamer basket over steaming water for 6 minutes (or microwave for 6 minutes).

Heat the oil in a medium-size skillet over medium heat and cook the onion and bell pepper, stirring occasionally, until softened, about 5 minutes. Add the potato and cook, stirring to combine, for another 2 minutes.

Whisk the eggs together in a bowl with the parsley, salt, and pepper. Pour the eggs over the vegetables in the skillet, cover, and cook gently over low heat for 8 minutes. Remove the lid and place under the preheated broiler to cook for 1 minute or until the top is set. Cut into wedges to serve.

SERVING IDEAS: You can serve wedges of tortilla de patatas warm or cold (it keeps well, covered and chilled, for 1 to 2 days).

For a Spanish-style meal, start with a bowl of Gazpacho (page 244) and accompany the tortilla with a salad and crusty bread.

Chakchouka

A colorful and spicy Tunisian vegetable and egg dish that makes a tasty and healthy breakfast or light lunch.

SERVES 4

3 tablespoons extra-virgin olive oil
1 red onion, diced
1 large red bell pepper, julienned
1 large green bell pepper, julienned
2 cloves garlic, finely chopped
1 small red chile, deseeded and finely chopped (or $\frac{1}{2}$ teaspoon chili powder)
1 teaspoon cumin
1 teaspoon paprika
1 teaspoon salt
14 ounces (420 g) canned whole tomatoes, chopped
4 large eggs

Heat the oil in a large skillet over medium heat and cook the onion, stirring, for 2 minutes. Add the bell peppers, garlic, and chile and cook, stirring regularly, for 10 minutes. Add the cumin, paprika, salt, and tomatoes, mix well, and simmer gently until thickened, about 10 minutes. Make four indentations in the mixture with the back of a spoon, and crack one egg into each. Cover and simmer until the eggs are set, about 5 minutes. Serve with crusty bread or lightly buttered whole-grain toast on the side.

Italian-Style Scrambled Eggs

Soft, creamy scrambled eggs combined with a selection of Italian-style vegetables and Parmesan cheese.

SERVES 4

8 large eggs
4 tablespoons milk
1 teaspoon sea salt
$\frac{1}{2}$ teaspoon freshly ground black pepper
2 tablespoons extra-virgin olive oil

1 onion, finely chopped

½ red bell pepper, finely diced

1 zucchini (courgette), finely chopped

4 tablespoons grated Parmesan cheese

8 slices of lightly buttered whole-grain toast, for serving

In a bowl, whisk the eggs, milk, salt, and pepper together gently.

Heat the olive oil in a large skillet over medium heat until lightly sizzling. Add the onion, bell pepper, and zucchini and cook, stirring occasionally, until the vegetables are softened, about 8 minutes. Reduce the heat to medium low, add the egg mixture, and cook, stirring continuously, until the eggs are barely set, about 2 minutes. Stir in the Parmesan cheese and cook until the eggs are creamy, about 30 seconds more. Remove from the heat and serve with slices of lightly buttered whole-grain toast.

► Sardine Toast Topper

Sardines are the perfect match with lemon juice and capers and make a great breakfast spread on hot buttered toast (lightly buttered, of course). Not only are sardines rich in healthy omega-3s, by including their delicate calcium-rich bones, sardines also help promote strong bones and teeth.

SERVES 4

8 ounces (240 g) canned sardines in water or oil, drained

4 teaspoons freshly squeezed lemon juice

4 teaspoons capers, rinsed and drained

1 teaspoon salt

½ teaspoon freshly ground black pepper

8 slices of whole-grain bread, toasted and lightly buttered

4 lemon wedges, for serving

Mash together the sardines, lemon juice, capers, salt, and pepper in a bowl until well combined. Spread equal amounts of the mixture over the pieces of lightly buttered toast and serve with lemon wedges for drizzling.

Creamy Fruit and Nut Oatmeal

A bowl of this creamy oatmeal sprinkled with dried fruits and nuts makes a warming and sustaining breakfast.

SERVES 4

5 cups cold water
2 cups rolled oats
½ teaspoon salt
½ teaspoon cinnamon
Cold milk, for serving
Brown sugar or honey, for serving
½ cup chopped dried fruit (such as raisins, figs, or apricots), for serving
4 tablespoons chopped nuts (such as walnuts, hazelnuts, or almonds)

Combine the water, oats, salt, and cinnamon in a saucepan. Bring to a boil over medium-high heat, stirring regularly to avoid lumps. Reduce the heat to medium and simmer for 10 minutes, stirring occasionally, until thick and creamy. Serve in bowls with milk, a little brown sugar or honey, and sprinkled with the fruit and nuts.

Raisin, Apricot, and Almond Muesli

One of the quickest and tastiest breakfasts is muesli. And because muesli typically contains a mixture of rolled oats (which are a whole grain), dried fruit, and nuts, it also makes a healthy start to the day. This recipe makes the equivalent of a large box of breakfast cereal.

MAKES 13 CUPS

8 cups of Wheaties (also known as Weeties in some countries)
4 cups rolled oats
½ cup raisins
½ cup sliced almonds
½ cup chopped dried apricots
½ cup desiccated or shredded unsweetened coconut

In a very large bowl combine the Wheaties, rolled oats, raisins, almonds, apricots, and coconut. Mix together thoroughly and store in an airtight container.

Smoked Salmon and Avocado Bagels

Because bagels are boiled and then baked, they have an appealing chewy texture. In this version, we use creamy avocado in place of the traditional cream cheese for a luscious heart-healthy alternative.

SERVES 4

2 avocados, peeled
4 teaspoons freshly squeezed lemon juice
Sea salt and freshly ground black pepper to taste
4 bagels (regular or whole grain), split in half and lightly toasted
7 ounces (200 g) sliced smoked salmon
24 capers, rinsed and drained
2 tablespoons finely chopped red onion

Mash the avocado in a bowl using a fork, add the lemon juice, and season with salt and pepper. Spread the toasted bagel halves with equal amounts of the avocado mixture.

Arrange the smoked salmon, capers, and red onion evenly on top and serve.

Italian-Style Pan-Fried Sandwich

A simple toasted sandwich with an Italian twist.

8 slices whole-grain bread
4 thin slices ham
3 ounces (90 g) thinly sliced mozzarella cheese
2 tomatoes, thinly sliced
4 teaspoons finely chopped fresh basil
Sea salt and freshly ground black pepper to taste
8 teaspoons extra-virgin olive oil
2 cloves garlic, peeled and cut in half

Top four slices of bread evenly with ham, cheese, tomatoes, and basil, and season with salt and pepper. Cover with the other four bread slices and lightly brush the sandwiches on both sides with the oil.

Heat a large skillet over medium heat and place the sandwiches into the pan (wait until the pan is hot before you add the sandwiches or else they'll stick). Cook for 2 minutes on each side, or until golden brown. Remove from the skillet, rub one side of each sandwich with the cut side of the garlic, and cut in half to serve.

VARIATIONS: Add rings of thinly sliced onion or a few sliced olives.

Replace the basil with a smear of pesto or use finely chopped sun-dried tomatoes instead of fresh.

Appetizers

Garlic Shrimp

A sizzling dish of shrimp flavored with fresh garlic, sea salt, and parsley and served with lemon wedges. Perfect as an appetizer on its own or served as part of a selection of tapas.

SERVES 4

4 tablespoons extra-virgin olive oil
24 large uncooked shrimp (prawns), peeled and deveined with bottom of tail left intact
4 cloves garlic, finely chopped
1 teaspoon sea salt
2 teaspoons finely chopped fresh flat-leaf parsley
Lemon wedges, for serving

Heat the oil in a large skillet over medium heat and add the shrimp, garlic, and salt. Cook, tossing regularly, about 3 minutes. Sprinkle with parsley and serve with lemon wedges for squeezing.

VARIATION: To make Chile-Garlic Shrimp, add 2 small fresh red chiles, deseeded and finely chopped, with the garlic and shrimp.

Lemongrass and Chile Mussels

Steamed mussels infused with classic Thai-style seasonings.

SERVES 4

1 cup coconut milk
2 scallions (white and green parts), thinly sliced on the diagonal
4 teaspoons finely chopped fresh lemongrass
4 teaspoons finely grated fresh ginger
2 small red chiles, deseeded and finely diced
2 cloves garlic, finely chopped
32 fresh mussels, cleaned and debearded
Cilantro (fresh coriander) leaves, for garnish

Place the coconut milk, scallions, lemongrass, ginger, chiles, and garlic in a large saucepan over high heat and bring to a boil. Add the mussels, cover the pot, and steam over low heat, shaking the pan occasionally, until the mussels open, about 5 minutes. Transfer the mussels to serving bowls, reserving the liquid in the pan. Heat the reserved liquid over high heat until reduced by half, about 3 minutes. Pour the liquid over the mussels and garnish with the cilantro leaves to serve.

TIP: Before cooking, discard any mussels with cracked shells. After cooking, discard any mussels that haven't opened.

▶ MediterrAsian Oysters

A succulent combination of Mediterranean-seasoned and Asian-seasoned oysters on the half shell. This dish is very easy to whip up and can be enjoyed as an appetizer or served as part of a seafood platter.

SERVES 4

Crushed ice, for serving
24 very fresh raw oysters on the half shell

MEDITERRANEAN DRESSING
2 tablespoons extra-virgin olive oil
2 tablespoons freshly squeezed lemon juice
4 teaspoons minced fresh flat-leaf parsley, plus sprigs for serving
2 teaspoons minced red onion
Pinch of freshly ground black pepper

ASIAN DRESSING
2 tablespoons fish sauce
2 tablespoons freshly squeezed lime juice
4 teaspoons minced cilantro (fresh coriander), plus sprigs for serving
2 teaspoons minced red chile
2 teaspoons minced scallion, white part only

Place the crushed ice on a large serving plate and arrange the oysters evenly over the top.

Mix together all the Mediterranean dressing ingredients in one bowl and all the Asian dressing ingredients in another bowl. Drizzle half the oysters with the Mediterranean dressing and the other half with the Asian dressing. Garnish with a sprig of parsley or cilantro and serve immediately

Asparagus with Garlic and Toasted Almonds

Fresh asparagus spears are sautéed in olive oil, seasoned with white wine, garlic, sea salt, and freshly ground pepper, and then scattered with freshly toasted sliced almonds. This makes an appetizing side dish. It can be served as an antipasto, meze, or tapas dish or served cold as a salad.

SERVES 4

½ cup sliced almonds
4 tablespoons extra-virgin olive oil
1 red onion, finely diced
24 asparagus spears, woody ends removed
2 cloves garlic, minced
1 teaspoon sea salt
½ teaspoon freshly ground black pepper
4 tablespoons dry white wine

Toast the almonds lightly in a skillet over medium heat until golden, 3 to 5 minutes. Remove and set aside.

Heat 3 tablespoons of the olive oil in the skillet over medium heat and cook the onion, stirring, for 3 minutes. Add the asparagus, garlic, salt, and pepper and cook, stirring regularly, for 2 minutes. Add the wine, cover the pan, and cook for 4 minutes. Add the toasted almonds, mix thoroughly, and serve on a plate drizzled with the remaining tablespoon of olive oil.

Fava Bean Puree with Pita Wedges

The vibrant green color and scrumptious flavor of the fava bean puree is a perfect combination with crisp baked pita wedges.

SERVES 4

4 medium-size whole-grain pita breads
4 cups frozen fava (broad) beans, cooked in boiling water for 5 minutes, rinsed under cold water, and skins removed
6 tablespoons extra-virgin olive oil

2 tablespoons freshly squeezed lemon juice
2 cloves garlic, minced
1 teaspoon sea salt
½ teaspoon freshly ground black pepper

Preheat the oven to 450°F (230°C).

Cut each pita bread into 8 wedges. Place on a baking tray and bake for 5 minutes.

While the pita wedges are baking, place the cooked fava beans, olive oil, lemon juice, garlic, salt, and pepper in a food processor or blender and process until smooth, scraping the sides occasionally. Spoon the puree into a small bowl and serve with the toasted pita wedges.

▶ Fava Beans with Marinated Artichoke Hearts and Olives

A tasty Greek meze (appetizer) dish with succulent kalamata olives, tender fava beans, and marinated artichoke hearts.

SERVES 4

3 cups frozen fava (broad) beans
32 kalamata olives
4 jarred marinated artichoke hearts, quartered
4 tablespoons extra-virgin olive oil
2 tablespoons freshly squeezed lemon juice
1 clove garlic, minced
1 teaspoon sea salt
4 teaspoons finely chopped fresh flat-leaf parsley
Freshly ground black pepper

Cook the fava beans in rapidly boiling water for 4 minutes, then rinse under cold water. Remove the leathery outer skin from the fava beans and discard. Mix together the shelled fava beans, olives, and artichoke hearts in a bowl.

Mix together the olive oil, lemon juice, garlic, and sea salt in a small bowl. Place equal amounts of the fava bean mixture on serving plates. Drizzle with the dressing, and top with the parsley and a little freshly ground black pepper.

Thai Fish Cakes with Sweet Chili Sauce

Fish cakes are a popular appetizer and snack in Thailand. In this recipe, delicately spiced fish cakes are served with sweet chili sauce for dipping.

SERVES 4

20 ounces (600 g) roughly chopped firm whitefish fillets
3 teaspoons Thai red curry paste
4 tablespoons cornstarch
2 tablespoon fish sauce
2 large egg whites
2 cloves garlic, minced
4 *kaffir* lime leaves (or 2 teaspoons of finely chopped lime zest)
2 scallions (white and green parts), trimmed and thinly sliced
4 tablespoons canola or peanut oil
Sweet chili sauce, for serving

Place the chopped fish fillets in a food processor or blender and pulse until smooth. Add the red curry paste, cornstarch, fish sauce, egg whites, and garlic and pulse until well combined. Transfer the fish mixture to a bowl, add the kaffir lime leaves and scallions, and stir to combine. Cover and refrigerate for 15 minutes.

Divide the mixture into 12 equal portions and shape each with wet hands into flat round patties. Heat 2 tablespoons of the oil in a large skillet over medium heat. Cook 6 fish cakes at a time, until golden brown, about 3 minutes per side. Remove to a serving plate and cook the remaining 6 fish cakes in the remaining 2 tablespoons of oil. Serve the fish cakes warm or at room temperature with sweet chili sauce for dipping.

Asian-Style Corn Fritters

These tasty fritters are delicious served with dipping sauces such as Nuoc Cham and Chinese-Style Dipping sauces.

4 cups corn kernels, preferably fresh
2 cups self-rising flour
4 scallions (white and green parts), trimmed and thinly sliced
2 large eggs, lightly beaten
4 tablespoons finely chopped cilantro (fresh coriander), plus sprigs for garnish
2 tablespoons fish sauce
2 teaspoons red curry paste mixed with 2 teaspoons boiling water
2 teaspoons salt
1 teaspoon ground black pepper
6 tablespoons canola or peanut oil
Thinly sliced cucumber, for garnish
Nuoc Cham Dipping Sauce (page 284), for serving
Chinese-Style Dipping Sauce (page 288), for serving

In a bowl, mix together the corn, flour, scallions, eggs, cilantro, fish sauce, curry paste, salt, and pepper until well combined. Shape the mixture into fritters using wet hands to prevent sticking.

Heat a large skillet over medium heat, add half the oil, and swirl to coat the surface. Cook half the fritters for 3 minutes each side, then remove from the pan and keep warm. Heat the remaining oil in the same pan and cook the other fritters. Garnish the fritters with sliced cucumber and sprigs of fresh cilantro. Serve with the dipping sauce of your choice.

VARIATION: To make shrimp fritters, replace the corn kernels with 2 cups of chopped cooked and peeled shrimp.

Spinach and Feta Parcels

A seasoned blend of spinach and feta cheese encased in light and flaky phyllo pastry. These delicate parcels can be served hot or cold as an appetizer, and they make great party finger food.

SERVES 4

5 tablespoons olive oil
1 onion, finely chopped
1 bunch spinach, stems removed and leaves chopped
1 tablespoon finely chopped fresh flat-leaf parsley
½ teaspoon dried oregano
½ teaspoon salt
¼ teaspoon freshly ground black pepper
3 ounces (100 g) feta cheese, crumbled
2 tablespoons butter, melted
1 package frozen phyllo (filo) pastry, thawed

Preheat the oven to 350°F (180°C).

Heat 2 tablespoons of the oil in a skillet over medium heat. Cook the onion, stirring, until softened, about 5 minutes. Add the spinach and cook, stirring regularly, for 3 minutes. Stir in the parsley, oregano, salt, and pepper and remove from the heat. Stir in the crumbled feta, combine well, and set aside to cool.

Combine the remaining 3 tablespoons of oil with the melted butter in a small bowl. Remove the phyllo pastry sheets from the package and, using a sharp knife or scissors, cut the dough lengthwise into 2½-inch-wide strips. Cover the strips of dough with a clean damp dishcloth to keep them from drying out and becoming brittle. Place 1 strip on a flat, clean surface and brush lightly with the melted butter and oil, then place a level tablespoon of the spinach and feta filling at one end. Fold the end of the strip over the filling at a 45-degree angle so that it forms a triangle. Continue folding, like you're folding a flag, until you have a completely sealed triangular-shaped parcel. Brush the outside lightly with the melted butter and oil. Repeat the entire process until you have used up all the spinach and feta filling (makes around 20 parcels). Arrange the parcels on a lightly greased baking tray and bake for 25 minutes. Serve hot or cold.

Sauces, Dips, and Spreads

Pesto Genoese

Pesto is one of the best-known and most versatile sauces of the Mediterranean region. This classic Genoese pesto is made with fresh basil, pine nuts, Parmesan cheese, garlic, and extra-virgin olive oil. Traditionally, pesto is made by grinding the ingredients together with a mortar and pestle; however, it's much quicker just to whip it up in a food processor or blender.

MAKES 1 CUP

1 cup tightly packed fresh basil
1/3 cup freshly grated Parmesan cheese
1/3 cup pine nuts, lightly toasted
1 clove garlic, roughly chopped
2 tablespoons water
1/2 teaspoon sea salt
1/4 teaspoon freshly ground black pepper
1/3 cup extra-virgin olive oil

In a food processor or blender, combine the basil, Parmesan, pine nuts, garlic, water, salt, and pepper. While you process, slowly pour the olive oil into the mix until all the ingredients turn into a smooth paste (you may have to scrape the sides occasionally). Store in the refrigerator, covered, for up to 3 days, or in the freezer for up to 3 months.

SERVING IDEAS: Pesto has a myriad of uses, such as tossed with hot pasta, spread over bruschetta, used as a pizza sauce, stirred into soups like minestrone just before serving, mixed with mayonnaise to dress salads and sandwiches, or served as a dip with vegetable crudités.

VARIATION: Walnuts, pistachios, macadamias, almonds, or cashews can be substituted for the pine nuts.

Sun-Dried Tomato and Walnut Pesto

A deliciously different pesto made with walnuts and richly flavored sun-dried tomatoes. You can use this pesto as a dip or spread, you can stir it into soups to add richness and flavor, and of course you can serve it with pasta.

MAKES 1 CUP

1 cup tightly packed fresh basil leaves
1/3 cup freshly grated Parmesan cheese
1/3 cup walnuts
6 oil-packed sun-dried tomatoes, roughly chopped
1 large clove garlic, roughly chopped
2 tablespoons water
1/2 teaspoon sea salt
1/4 teaspoon freshly ground black pepper
1/3 cup extra-virgin olive oil

In a food processor, combine the basil, Parmesan, walnuts, sun-dried tomatoes, garlic, water, salt, and pepper. While you process, slowly pour the olive oil into the mix until all the ingredients turn into a smooth paste (you may have to scrape the sides occasionally). Store in the refrigerator, covered, for up to 3 days, or in the freezer for up to 3 months.

VARIATION: Pine nuts, pistachio nuts, macadamias, almonds, or cashews can be substituted for the walnuts.

Asian Cilantro-Peanut Pesto

This Asian-inspired pesto makes an enticing change from traditional pesto and is wonderful tossed through Asian noodles with vegetables and seafood or chicken.

MAKES 1 CUP

1 cup tightly packed cilantro (fresh coriander)
⅓ cup unsalted roasted peanuts
1 small green chile, deseeded and roughly chopped
1 clove garlic, roughly chopped
1 teaspoon finely grated fresh ginger
2 tablespoons freshly squeezed lime juice
1 tablespoon fish sauce
½ tablespoon brown sugar
½ teaspoon salt
⅓ cup peanut oil

In a food processor or blender, combine the cilantro, peanuts, chile, garlic, ginger, lime juice, fish sauce, sugar, and salt. While you process, slowly pour the peanut oil into the mix until all the ingredients turn into a smooth paste (you may have to scrape the sides occasionally). Store in the refrigerator, covered, for up to 3 days, or in the freezer for up to 3 months.

▶ Tapenade

Tapenade is a luscious Provençal paste made with olives, olive oil, anchovies, capers, and garlic. Traditionally, it's made using a mortar and pestle, but to save time and energy you can get similar results by using a food processor.

MAKES ½ CUP

1 clove garlic, roughly chopped
1 tablespoon freshly squeezed lemon juice
2 tablespoons extra-virgin olive oil
¾ cup pitted black olives
1 tablespoon capers
2 anchovy fillets
¼ teaspoon freshly ground black pepper

Place all ingredients in a food processor or blender and process until smooth. Store in the refrigerator, covered, for up to 3 days, or in the freezer for up to 3 months.

SERVING IDEAS: Tapenade can be used to season grilled fish or chicken; it's delicious spread on sliced baguette and topped with chopped tomatoes; or simply serve it with crackers or crusty bread and vegetable crudités for dipping.

▶ Raita

The combination of cucumber and yogurt makes a traditional cooling accompaniment to serve with spicy Indian dishes such as South Indian Shrimp Curry (page 174) or Fragrant Chicken Curry (page 176).

MAKES 1½ CUPS

1 cup plain thick yogurt (Greek-style yogurt is best)
½ cup finely chopped cucumber, peeled and deseeded
½ clove garlic, minced
2 teaspoons freshly squeezed lemon juice
½ teaspoon salt

In a small bowl, mix together the yogurt, cucumber, garlic, lemon juice, and salt until well combined. Store in the refrigerator, covered, for up to 2 days.

Indonesian Peanut Sauce

This mouthwatering peanut sauce has a rich, nutty flavor and a delightful creamy texture. It makes an ideal dipping sauce for satay (marinated and grilled chicken, meat, or seafood skewers) and a pouring sauce for the classic Indonesian salad Gado Gado (page 259).

MAKES 2 CUPS

1 tablespoon canola or peanut oil
2 cloves garlic, finely chopped
½ teaspoon shrimp paste (or 1 tablespoon fish sauce)
1 cup coconut milk
1 cup water
6 tablespoons natural peanut butter
4 tablespoons soy sauce
4 teaspoons brown sugar
½ teaspoon *sambal oelek* (Indonesian chili sauce), or ¼ teaspoon chili powder
1 tablespoon freshly squeezed lemon juice

Heat the oil in a skillet over medium heat. Add the garlic and shrimp paste and cook, stirring constantly to dissolve the shrimp paste, for 1 minute. Add the coconut milk, water, peanut butter, soy sauce, sugar, and sambal oelek and bring to a boil. Reduce the heat and simmer, stirring regularly, until the sauce reaches a creamy consistency, 10 to 12 minutes. Add the lemon juice, and stir to combine. Store in the refrigerator, covered, for up to 3 days, or in the freezer for up to 3 months.

Romesco Sauce

A robust Spanish sauce made from a pureed mix of grilled red peppers, toasted almonds, garlic, chile, red wine vinegar, and olive oil. This delicious and versatile sauce can be drizzled over grilled fish, chicken, seafood, or vegetables; used as a salad dressing, dip, or spread; stirred into stews to add richness and color; and it makes a wonderful pasta sauce.

MAKES 1 CUP

1 red bell pepper, deseeded and quartered
½ cup sliced almonds
⅓ cup extra-virgin olive oil
2 tablespoons red wine vinegar
1 tablespoon water
1 clove garlic, roughly chopped
1 small red chile, deseeded and chopped (or ½ teaspoon chili powder)
½ teaspoon salt
¼ teaspoon freshly ground black pepper

Place the bell pepper (skin side up) under a hot oven broiler (griller) until the skin blackens all over, about 10 minutes. Remove and cover the charred pepper with a clean dishcloth or plastic wrap for 5 minutes to allow the steam to loosen the skin from the pepper flesh.

While the pepper cools, place the almonds in a frying pan and toast over a gentle heat, stirring regularly so they don't burn, until golden brown.

Peel off the blackened skin from the pepper and roughly cut the flesh into pieces. In a blender or food processor, combine the roasted pepper, toasted almonds, oil, vinegar, water, garlic, chile, salt, and pepper and blend until smooth. Store in the refrigerator, covered, for up to 3 days, or in the freezer for up to 3 months.

Nuoc Cham Dipping Sauce

This delicious, sweet, and spicy Vietnamese dipping sauce is the perfect accompaniment to Vietnamese rice paper rolls or any Asian-style finger food.

MAKES ½ CUP

2 tablespoons water
1 tablespoon sugar
2 tablespoons freshly squeezed lemon juice
2 tablespoons fish sauce
2 tablespoons rice vinegar
1 clove garlic, minced
1 red chile, deseeded and finely chopped

Mix together the water and sugar in a small bowl until dissolved. Stir in the lemon juice, fish sauce, vinegar, garlic, and chile until well combined. Store in the refrigerator, covered, for up to 1 week.

TIP: In this nuoc cham recipe we have purposely made the sauce milder, heat-wise, by finely chopping the chile. Traditionally the chile and other ingredients are ground with a mortar and pestle, which makes the sauce hotter. Feel free to do this if you like, or you can process all the ingredients in a blender (however, this tends to make the nuoc cham go frothy).

Hummus

Hummus is a creamy puree of chickpeas and tahini (sesame seed paste) seasoned with lemon juice and garlic, and it is a popular spread and dip in Greece and throughout the Middle East. Hummus can be served as part of a meze platter; with bread or vegetable crudités for dipping; as a spread or filling for pita, lavash, or Turkish *pide* bread; or as a tasty, creamy alternative to butter in sandwiches. A spoonful or two can also be added to Middle Eastern or Greek-style pilafs and stews to add richness.

MAKES 2 CUPS

14 ounces (420 g) canned chickpeas (garbanzo beans), rinsed and drained
½ cup tahini (sesame paste)

¼ cup freshly squeezed lemon juice
¼ cup water
2 cloves garlic, roughly chopped
1 teaspoon sea salt

Place all ingredients in a food processor or blender and process until smooth, scraping the sides occasionally. Store in the refrigerator, covered, for up to 1 week, or the freezer for up to 3 months.

VARIATION: If you like a spicier hummus, add a small red chile (chopped) or a pinch of cayenne pepper, or try a little cumin for a more exotic version.

▶ Salsa Verde

Made from a mixture of fresh herbs, capers, and anchovies, this piquant Italian green sauce can be served as a no-cook pasta sauce (such as Pasta with Salsa Verde and Smoked Salmon, page 152), with grilled fish or chicken, or tossed with cooked potatoes for a Mediterranean-style potato salad.

MAKES ½ CUP

4 anchovy fillets, finely chopped
4 tablespoons extra-virgin olive oil
3 tablespoons finely chopped fresh flat-leaf parsley
3 tablespoons finely chopped fresh basil
2 tablespoons freshly squeezed lemon juice
1 scallion (white and green parts), trimmed and finely chopped
1 tablespoon capers, rinsed, drained, and finely chopped
1 clove garlic, minced
½ teaspoon sea salt
¼ teaspoon freshly ground black pepper

Mix together all ingredients in a bowl until well combined. Store in the refrigerator, covered, for up to 2 days.

Baba Ghanoush

The smoky flavor and creamy texture of this Middle Eastern eggplant puree is truly unique and absolutely delectable. It's wonderful served as a dip or a spread.

MAKES 1 CUP

1 large eggplant (aubergine), cut in half lengthways
2 tablespoons freshly squeezed lemon juice
2 tablespoons tahini (sesame paste)
2 tablespoons extra-virgin olive oil
1 clove garlic, roughly chopped
1 teaspoon sea salt
½ teaspoon ground black pepper

Preheat an oven broiler (griller). Place the eggplant halves, skin side up, on a baking tray (or line the broiler tray with foil). Cook the eggplant about 1 inch from the heat source for 20 minutes. Remove the eggplant and let it cool to room temperature.

Scoop out the eggplant flesh from the skin with a spoon, and place in a food processor or blender with the lemon juice, tahini, oil, garlic, salt, and pepper; process until smooth. Store in the refrigerator, covered, for up to 3 days, or in the freezer for up to 3 months.

Good-quality store-bought mayonnaise can be blended with different ingredients to create a range of flavorful sauces. The following suggestions are delicious spread on bread, transforming simple sandwiches and burgers into gourmet fare. They are versatile and can be served as an accompaniment with many other dishes.

Aioli. Mix together 4 tablespoons mayonnaise with 1 clove minced garlic and 2 teaspoons extra-virgin olive oil. This easy version of traditional Provençal garlic mayonnaise makes a delicious accompaniment with cooked fish and shellfish, roast chicken, or a selection of boiled eggs, potatoes, raw and cooked vegetables, and bread.

Dijon Mayonnaise. Mix together 4 tablespoons of mayonnaise with 2 teaspoons Dijon mustard.

Pesto Mayonnaise. Mix together 4 tablespoons mayonnaise with 2 tablespoons Pesto Genoese (page 278).

Wasabi Mayonnaise. Mix together 4 tablespoons mayonnaise with 2 teaspoons wasabi paste.

Lime Mayonnaise. Mix together 4 tablespoons mayonnaise with 2 tablespoons freshly squeezed lime juice (great with seafood).

Sweet Chili Mayonnaise. Mix together 4 tablespoons mayonnaise with 2 tablespoons sweet chili sauce.

Curry Mayonnaise. Mix together 4 tablespoons mayonnaise with 1 teaspoon curry powder.

Seafood Sauce. Mix together 4 tablespoons mayonnaise with 4 teaspoons ketchup, 1 teaspoon of freshly squeezed lemon juice, and salt and pepper to taste.

Chinese-Style Dipping Sauce

This is a good dipping sauce for Chinese-Style Chicken and Vegetable Rolls (page 213) and Asian-Style Corn Fritters (page 275).

MAKES ³/₄ CUP

½ cup chicken stock
2 tablespoons soy sauce
2 teaspoons Chinese rice wine
1 teaspoon sesame oil
1 teaspoon finely grated fresh ginger
½ clove garlic, crushed
1 teaspoon sugar

Mix together all ingredients in a small bowl until well combined. Store in the refrigerator, covered, for up to 3 days.

Sesame-Hoisin Dipping Sauce

The combination of thick, savory-sweet hoisin sauce with salty soy, nutty sesame oil, and a hint of garlic makes a heavenly dipping sauce to serve with rice paper rolls (page 211).

MAKES ¹/₃ CUP

3 tablespoons hoisin sauce
3 tablespoons soy sauce
2 tablespoons water
2 teaspoons sesame oil
½ clove garlic, minced

Mix together all ingredients in a small bowl until well combined. Store in the refrigerator, covered, for up to 1 week.

Italian Vinaigrette

A simple and flavorsome all-purpose dressing that is ideal with Italian-style salads.

MAKES ¼ CUP

2½ tablespoons extra-virgin olive oil
1½ tablespoons balsamic vinegar
½ clove garlic, minced
¼ teaspoon sea salt
¼ teaspoon freshly ground black pepper

Shake together all ingredients in a screw-top jar until well combined. Store in the refrigerator, covered, for up to 1 week.

Provençal Vinaigrette

This traditional dressing is a perfect match with Salade Niçoise (page 254) or a simple green salad.

MAKES ¼ CUP

3 tablespoons extra-virgin olive oil
1 tablespoon white wine vinegar
½ teaspoon Dijon mustard
½ clove garlic, minced
¼ teaspoon sea salt
¼ teaspoon freshly ground black pepper

Mix together all ingredients in a bowl until well combined. Store in the refrigerator, covered, for up to 1 week.

▶ Savory Salmon Spread

This easy-to-prepare omega-3-rich spread can be used as a sandwich or wrap filling, and it also makes a tasty whole-grain cracker topping.

14 ounces (420 g) canned Alaskan red salmon, bones removed
2 tablespoons mayonnaise
2 tablespoons extra-virgin olive oil
$1/2$ teaspoon salt
$1/2$ teaspoon freshly ground black pepper
$1^1/2$ tablespoons finely chopped red onion
1 tablespoon freshly squeezed lemon juice
1 tablespoon finely chopped fresh flat-leaf parsley
1 teaspoon finely chopped capers

Mash the salmon in a bowl with the mayonnaise, olive oil, salt, and pepper. Add the onion, lemon juice, parsley, and capers and mix thoroughly to combine. Store in the refrigerator, covered, for up to 3 days.

▶ Savory Tuna Spread

This versatile spread can be used as a sandwich filling or toast topping, spread on whole-grain crackers, served as part of a salad plate, or tossed through pasta.

14 ounces (420 g) canned tuna
2 tablespoons mayonnaise
2 tablespoons extra-virgin olive oil
$1/2$ teaspoon salt
$1/2$ teaspoon freshly ground black pepper
2 ripe tomatoes, diced
8 pitted black olives, finely chopped
$1^1/2$ tablespoons finely chopped red onion

Mash the tuna in a bowl with the mayonnaise, olive oil, salt, and pepper. Add the tomatoes, olives, and onion and mix thoroughly to combine. Store in the refrigerator, covered, for up to 3 days.

Desserts

Mixed Berry Coulis
with Greek Vanilla Yogurt

Fresh strawberries and blueberries are folded through a berry sauce and served with vanilla-flavored Greek-style yogurt (Greek yogurt is readily available in the United States and can't really be substituted with regular yogurt for this dessert) and almonds.

SERVES 4

16 ounces (480 g) strawberries, hulled
10 ounces (300 g) blueberries
4 tablespoons confectioners' sugar
¾ cup Greek-style yogurt
1 teaspoon vanilla extract
4 tablespoons sliced almonds (lightly toasted, if desired)

Put half the strawberries and half the blueberries in a blender with 2 tablespoons of the sugar, and process until smooth. Cut the remaining strawberries into quarters, toss with the remaining blueberries, then fold into the berry sauce. Mix together the yogurt, vanilla, and remaining sugar in a small bowl until well combined. Spoon the berry coulis into four dessert bowls, top with the vanilla yogurt, and scatter each with a tablespoon of almonds.

Fruit Couscous with
Honey-Cinnamon Yogurt

Orange-infused couscous with fresh strawberries, grapes, and a dollop of honey-cinnamon yogurt. Serve as a dessert or as a breakfast dish.

SERVES 4

1 cup freshly squeezed orange juice
¼ cup water
1 tablespoon sugar
1 cup couscous
2 cups red or white seedless grapes
2 cups sliced fresh strawberries

8 tablespoons thick natural-set yogurt (Greek yogurt is ideal)
2 tablespoons honey
½ teaspoon ground cinnamon

Heat the orange juice, water, and sugar in a saucepan over high heat until it comes to a boil. Place the couscous in a heatproof bowl, pour over the boiling liquid, and cover with a plate or clean dishcloth to trap the steam. After 5 minutes, fluff up the couscous with a fork, then stir in the grapes and sliced strawberries. Cover and cool in the fridge.

While the fruit couscous is cooling, mix together the yogurt, honey, and cinnamon in a bowl. Serve the fruit couscous with the honey-cinnamon yogurt drizzled on top and a dusting of more cinnamon, if you like.

VARIATION: Fresh sliced peaches and berries like raspberries and blackberries also go perfectly with this dessert.

▶ Mango with Lime Syrup and Toasted Coconut

A sweet and simple Thai dessert, perfect for cooling the palate after a hot Thai curry.

SERVES 4

½ cup water
4 tablespoons freshly squeezed lime juice
2 tablespoons sugar
2 teaspoons freshly grated lime zest
4 tablespoons shredded dried coconut
4 mangoes, peeled, seeds removed, and flesh cut into cubes

Combine the water, lime juice, sugar, and lime zest in a small saucepan, stir to combine, simmer gently for 5 minutes until reduced by about half, then strain to remove the zest.

Toast the coconut in a skillet over medium heat. Arrange the cubed mango on plates, drizzle with the lime syrup, and sprinkle with the toasted coconut to serve.

Pears with Peach Ricotta Whip and Almonds

Ricotta cheese makes the perfect base for this creamy fruit dessert.

SERVES 4

¾ cup ricotta cheese
¾ cup drained canned sliced peaches
1 tablespoon confectioners' sugar
12 canned pear halves
4 tablespoons sliced almonds

Place the ricotta cheese, peaches, and sugar in a food processor or blender and process for 1 minute. Pour the mixture into a bowl and chill, covered, in the refrigerator for 2 hours to firm (or in the freezer for 1 hour).

Put three pear halves in each serving bowl, pour over the peach ricotta whip, and sprinkle with the almonds.

Provençal Apple and Walnut Pie

This dessert tastes delicious served warm from the oven and topped with a scoop of good-quality vanilla ice cream.

SERVES 4

2 large egg whites
½ cup sugar
1 teaspoon vanilla extract
1 teaspoon baking powder
½ teaspoon cinnamon
½ cup all-purpose (plain) flour
1 cup peeled and diced apple
¼ cup chopped walnuts
Vanilla ice cream, for serving

Preheat the oven to 350°F (180°C), and lightly grease a pie plate.

Beat the eggs, sugar, vanilla, baking powder, and cinnamon in a bowl until light and fluffy. Mix in the flour until well blended, then stir in the apples and walnuts. Pour the mixture into the prepared pie plate and bake for 30 minutes. Serve cut in wedges and topped with a scoop of vanilla ice cream.

VARIATIONS: Replace the chopped apples with other soft fruit like berries, apricots, or peaches.

Use other chopped nuts like hazelnuts or almonds instead of walnuts.

This pie also tastes great served with custard.

Tunisian Orange, Date, and Pistachio Salad

Cinnamon adds an exotic touch to a plate of refreshing sliced oranges garnished with dates and pistachio nuts. Serve this simple dessert as is or with a scoop of ice cream or yogurt.

SERVES 4

8 oranges (6 oranges peeled and all the white pith removed with
   a sharp knife, and 2 oranges juiced)
2 teaspoons confectioners' sugar
$\frac{1}{2}$ teaspoon cinnamon
12 dried dates, finely chopped
20 pistachio nuts, peeled and chopped

Slice the peeled oranges into rounds and arrange, overlapping, in a shallow serving bowl. Combine the orange juice with the sugar and cinnamon. Drizzle the juice over the orange rounds and garnish with the chopped dates and pistachio nuts.

VARIATION: Replace the pistachio nuts with slivered almonds.

Asian-Style Fruit Salad

This exotic salad of fresh and canned fruits provides the perfect ending to any Asian meal (or any meal, for that matter).

SERVES 4

2 kiwi fruit, peeled and thinly sliced
2 mangoes, peeled, seeds removed, and flesh cut into cubes
2 mandarins, peeled and divided into segments
1 cup drained canned lychees
1 cup drained canned pineapple pieces
Ice cream, fresh or frozen yogurt, or sorbet, for serving

Combine all the fruits in a bowl and toss gently to mix. Serve with a scoop of ice cream, fresh or frozen yogurt, or sorbet.

VARIATION: A variety of tropical fruits, including bananas, watermelon, honeydew melon, papaya, cantaloupe, Asian pear (*nashi*), guavas, and passion fruit can be used in this Asian-inspired fruit salad.

Strawberries and Mascarpone Cheese

This dessert is simplicity itself.

SERVES 4

1 cup mascarpone cheese
2 tablespoons confectioners' sugar
28 fresh, ripe strawberries, hulled

Mix together the mascarpone cheese and sugar in a small bowl until well combined. Serve the strawberries with the sweetened mascarpone cheese for dipping.

VARIATIONS: Replace the mascarpone cheese with crème fraîche.

As an alternative, you can macerate the strawberries to allow them to soften: Remove the stems and cut the strawberries lengthwise into quarters. Toss them in a bowl with a little superfine or confectioners' sugar and dash of fruit liqueur like Cointreau. Cover and allow to macerate in the refrigerator for at least 1 hour.

Mango, Grape, and Honeydew Melon Salad

The luscious flesh of these fruits, which range in color from pale green to deep orange, makes a delicious fruit salad. Orange fruits are an excellent source of beta-carotene, a powerful antioxidant that converts in the body to vitamin A, which is important for healthy skin and good vision.

SERVES 4

2 cups red or green seedless grapes
4 mangoes, peeled, seeds removed, and flesh cut into cubes
1 honeydew melon, peeled and flesh cut into cubes
2 tablespoons sugar
4 tablespoons water
Ice cream, fresh or frozen yogurt, or sorbet, for serving

Combine all the fruits in a serving dish. Mix the sugar and water until dissolved and toss gently with the fruit to coat. Serve by itself or with a scoop of ice cream, fresh or frozen yogurt, or sorbet.

VARIATION: For a simple yet exotic warm fruit compote, combine the grapes, mango, and honeydew melon in a saucepan with 1 cup of either orange or pineapple juice, 2 tablespoons brown sugar, 6 drops of vanilla extract, and ¼ teaspoon cinnamon (add 4 tablespoons Cointreau or rum, if desired). Simmer gently, covered, for 10 minutes, stirring occasionally. Serve the warm compote topped with a scoop of ice cream, fresh or frozen yogurt, or sorbet for a refreshing temperature contrast.

Middle Eastern Fruit and Nut Compote

A simple but exotic Middle Eastern dessert in which dried fruits are simmered in a cinnamon-infused syrup until plump and tender.

SERVES 4

1 cup orange juice
½ cup water
1 tablespoon brown sugar
½ teaspoon cinnamon
1 cup dried apricots
½ cup dried figs
½ cup raisins
Ice cream or fresh or frozen yogurt, for serving
4 tablespoons toasted sliced almonds

Place the orange juice, water, sugar, and cinnamon in a small saucepan, stir to combine, and bring to a boil. Add the apricots, figs, and raisins; cover the pot; reduce the heat to medium-low; and simmer for 20 minutes. Serve the fruit compote in bowls with a spoonful of ice cream or yogurt and sprinkled with the almonds.

VARIATION: Other dried fruits like prunes, apples, and peaches can also be used, and pistachio nuts or pine nuts can be substituted for the almonds.

SELECT BIBLIOGRAPHY

UNLOCKING THE SECRETS OF THE
MEDITERRANEAN DIET AND THE ASIAN DIET

Campbell, T. C., and C. Junshi. "Diet and chronic degenerative diseases: Perspectives from China." *American Journal of Clinical Nutrition* 59, suppl. (1994):1153S–1161S.

Chau, P., et al. "Dietary habits, health beliefs, and food practices of elderly Chinese women." *Journal of the American Dietetic Association* 90:4 (1990):579–580.

Chen, J., et al. "Historical development of Chinese dietary patterns and nutrition from the ancient to the modern society." *World Review of Nutrition and Dietetics* 79 (1996):133–153.

Chen, J., T. C. Campbell, J. Li, and R. Peto. *Diet, Lifestyle and Mortality in China, a Study of the Characteristics of 65 Chinese Cantons*. Oxford, Ithaca, NY, and Beijing: Oxford University Press, Cornell University Press, and People's Republic Publishing House, 1990.

de Lorgeril, M., P. Salen, J. L. Martin, et al. "Effect of a Mediterranean-type of diet on the rate of cardiovascular complications in coronary patients: Insights into the cardioprotective effects of certain nutriments." *Journal of the American College of Cardiology* 28 (1996):1103–1108.

de Lorgeril, M. "The Mediterranean diet in the prevention of coronary heart disease." *Nutrition* 14 (1998):55–57.

Ferro-Luzzi, A., and F. Branca. "Mediterranean diet, Italian type: Prototype of a healthy diet." *American Journal of Clinical Nutrition* 61 (1995):1338S–1345S.

Ferro-Luzzi, A., and S. Sette. "The Mediterranean diet: An attempt to define its present and past composition." *European Journal of Clinical Nutrition* 43, Supplement 2 (1989):13–29.

Haber, B. "The Mediterranean diet: A view from history." *American Journal of Clinical Nutrition* 66 (1997):1053A–1057S.

Harvard School of Public Health. "Faculty Research: Mediterranean Diet Lengthens Life." December 1995, http://www.hsph.harvard.edu/around/dt.html.

Ishimoto, H., et al. "Epidemiological study on relationship between breast cancer mortality and dietary factors." *Tokushima Journal of Experimental Medecine* 41 (1994): 3–4, 103–114.

Kushi, L., et al. "Health implications of Mediterranean diets in light of contemporary knowledge: 1. Plant foods and dairy products." *American Journal of Clinical Nutrition* 61 (1995):1407S–1415S.

———. "Health implications of Mediterranean diets in light of contemporary knowledge: 2. Meat, wine, fats, and oils." *American Journal of Clinical Nutrition* 61 (1995):1416S–1427S.

Keys, A., C. Aravanis, H. Blackburn, R. Buzina, et al. *Seven Countries. A Multivariate Analysis of Death and Coronary Heart Disease*. Cambridge, MA: Harvard University Press, 1980.

Keys, A. "Mediterranean diet and public health: Personal reflections." *American Journal of Clinical Nutrition* 61 (1995):1321S–1323S.

Keys, A., A. Menotti, M. J. Karvonen, C. Aravanis, et al. "The diet and 15-year death rate in the Seven Countries Study." *American Journal of Epidemiology* 124(6) (1986):903–915.

Kolonel, L. N. "Variability in diet and its relation to risk in ethnic and migrant groups." *Basic Life Science* 43 (1988):129–135.

Kromhout, D., A. Keys, C. Aravanis, et al. "Food consumption patterns in the 1960s in seven countries." *American Journal of Clinical Nutrition* 49 (1989):889–894.

Lee, M. M., et al. "Case-control study of diet and prostate cancer in China." *Cancer Causes and Control* 6 (1998): 545–552.

Manousos, O., N. Day, D. Trichopoulos, F. Garovassilis, et al. "Diet and colorectal cancer: A case-control study in

Greece." *International Journal of Cancer* 32 (1983):1–5.

Nestle, M. "Mediterranean diets: Science and policy implications." *American Journal of Clinical Nutrition* 61, suppl. (1995):6.

Popkin, B. M., et al. "The nutrition transition in China: A cross-sectional analysis." *European Journal of Clinical Nutrition* 47 (1993):5, 333–346.

Renaud, S., et al. "Cretan Mediterranean diet for prevention of coronary artery disease." *American Journal of Clinical Nutrition* 62, suppl. (1995):1360S–1367S.

Shaper, A. G. "Reflections on the Seven Countries Study." *Lancet* 347 (1996):208.

Tavani, A., and C. La Vecchia. "Fruit and vegetable consumption and cancer risk in a Mediterranean population." *American Journal of Clinical Nutrition.* 61, suppl. (1995):1374S–1377S.

Tominaga, S., et al. "An ecological study on diet/nutrition and cancer in Japan." *International Journal of Cancer* 10, suppl. (1997):2–6.

"Traditional healthy Asian diet pyramid: Preliminary concept." http://www.cornell.edu/pyramid1.html

Trichopoulou, A., P. Lagiou, and D. Trichopoulos. "Traditional Greek diet and coronary heart disease." *Journal of Cardiovascular Risk* 1 (1994):9–15.

Verschuren, W. M. M., D. R. Jacobs, B. P. M. Bloemberg, et al. "Serum total cholesterol and long-term coronary heart disease mortality in different cultures: Twenty-five-year follow-up of the Seven Countries Study." *Journal of the American Medical Association* 274 (1995): 31–136.

Waterlow, J. C. "Diet of the classical period of Greece and Rome." *European Journal of Clinical Nutrition* 43 (1989): 3–12.

Whittemore, A. S., et al. "Diet, physical activity, and colorectal cancer among Chinese in North America and China." *Journal of the National Cancer Institute* 82 (1990):915–26.

Willett, W. C. "Diet and health: What should we eat?" *Science* 264 (1994):532–537.

Willett, W. C., F. Sacks, A. Trichopoulou, G. Drescher, et al. "Mediterranean Diet Pyramid: A Cultural Model for Healthy Eating." *American Journal of Clinical Nutrition* 61, suppl. (1995): 1402S–1406S.

FAT FUNDAMENTALS

Ascherio, A., C. H. Hennekens, J. E. Buring, C. Master, et al. "Trans-fatty acids intake and risk of myocardial infarction (heart attack)." *Circulation* 89 (1994):94–101.

Campbell, L., et al. "The high-monounsaturated fat diet as a practical alternative for NIDDM (Type II Diabetes)." *Diabetes Care* 17 (1994):177–182.

Cleland, L. G., and M. J. James. "Rheumatoid arthritis and the balance of dietary n-6 (omega-6) and n-3 (omega-3) essential fatty acids." *British Journal of Rheumatology* 36 (1997):513–514.

Cumming, R. G., and R. J. Klineberg. "Case-control study of risk factors for hip fractures in the elderly." *American Journal of Epidemiology* 139 (1994):493–505.

Derr, J., P. M. Kris-Etherton, T. A. Pearson, and F. H. Seligson. "The role of fatty acid saturation on plasma lipids, lipoproteins, and apolipoproteins: II. The plasma total and low-density lipoprotein cholesterol response of individual fatty acids." *Metabolism* 42 (1993):130–134.

Dreon, D. M., K. M. Vranizan, R. M. Krauss, M. A. Austin, et al. "The effects of polyunsaturated fat vs monounsaturated fat on plasma lipoproteins." *Journal of the American Medical Association* 263 (1990):2462–2466.

Feldman, B. "Assorted monounsaturated fatty acids promote healthy hearts." *American Journal of Clinical Nutrition* 70 (1999):953–954.

Feskanich, D., W. C. Willet, M. J. Stampfer, and G. A. Colditz. "Milk, dietary calcium, and bone fractures in women: a 12-year prospective study." *American Journal of Public Health* 87 (1997):992–997.

Gardner, C. D., and H. C. Kraemer. "Monounsaturated versus polyunsaturated dietary fat and serum lipids. A meta-analysis." *Arteriosclerosis, Thrombosis, and Vascular Biology* 15 (1995):1917–1927.

Gerber, M., and S. Richardson. "Consumption of olive oil and specific food groups in relation to breast cancer risk in Greece." *Journal of the National Cancer Institute* 87(13) (1995):1021–1022.

Grundy, S. M. "Monounsaturated fatty acids, plasma cholesterol, and coronary heart disease." *American Journal of Clinical Nutrition* 45 (1987):1168–1175.

Haas, C. "Barley, the olive and wine, dietary and therapeutic triad of ancient Mediterranean people." *Annales de Medecine Interne* (Paris) 149(5) (1998):275–279.

Huang, Z., J. H. Himes, and P. G. McGovern. "Nutrition and subsequent hip fracture risk among a national cohort of white women." *American Journal of Epidemiology* 144 (1996):124–134.

Hu, F. B., M. J. Stampfer, J. E. Manson, E. Rimm, et al. "Dietary fat intake and the risk of coronary heart disease in women." *New England Journal of Medicine* 337 (1997):21,1491–1499.

Judd, J. T., B. A. Clevidence, R. A. Muesing, J. Wittes, et al. "Dietary trans fatty acids: Effects of plasma lipids and lipoproteins on healthy men and women." *American Journal of Clinical Nutrition* 59 (1994):861–868.

Katan, M., R. P. Mensink, and P. L. Zock. "Trans fatty acids and their effect on lipoproteins in humans." *Annual Review of Nutrition* 15 (1995):473–493.

Kris-Etherton, P. M. "Monounsaturated fatty acids and risk of cardiovascular disease." *Circulation* 100 (1999): 1253–1258.

Kris-Etherton, P. M., T. A. Pearson, Y. Wan, R. L. Hargrove, et al. "High-monounsaturated fatty acid diets lower both plasma cholesterol and triacylglycerol concentrations." *American Journal of Clinical Nutrition* 70 (1999):1009–1015.

Larsen, L. F., J. Jespersen, and P. Marckmann. "Are olive oil diets antithrombotic? Diets enriched with olive, rapeseed, or sunflower oil affect postprandial factor VII differently." *American Journal of Clinical Nutrition* 70(6) (1999):976–982.

Linos, A., V. G. Kaklamani, E. Kaklamani, Y. Koumantaki, et al. "Dietary factors in relation to rheumatoid arthritis: a role for olive oil and cooked vegetables?" *American Journal of Clinical Nutrition* 70(6) (1999):1077–1082.

Mata, P., J. A. Garrido, J. M. Ordovas, et al. "Effect of dietary monounsaturated fatty acids on plasma lipoproteins and apolipoproteins in women." *American Journal of Clinical Nutrition* 56 (1992):77–83.

Mattson, F. H., and S. M. Grundy. "Comparison of effects of dietary saturated, monounsaturated, and polyunsaturated fatty acids on plasma lipids and lipoproteins in man." *Journal of Lipid Research* 26 (1985):94–202.

Massaro, M., M. A. Carluccio, and R. De Caterina. "Direct vascular antiatherogenic effects of oleic acid: A clue to the cardioprotective effects of the Mediterranean diet." *Cardiologia* 44(6) (1999):507–513.

Mensink, R. P., and M. B. Katan. "Effect of a dietary fatty acids on serum lipids and lipoproteins—a meta-analysis of 27 trials." *Arteriosclerosis, Thrombosis, and Vascular Biology* 12 (1992):911–919.

Parthasarathy, S. J., J. C. Khoo, J. E. Miller, J. Barnett, et al. "Low density lipoprotein enriched in oleic acid is protected against oxidative modification: Implication for dietary prevention of atherosclerosis." *Proceedings of the National Academy of Sciences* 87 (1990):3894–3898.

Reid, D. M., and S. A. New. "Nutritional influences on bone mass." *Proceedings of the Nutrition Society* 56 (1997): 977–987.

Sacks, F. M., and W. C. Willet. "Chewing the fat: how much and what kind." *New England Journal of Medicine* 324 (1991):121–123.

———. "More on chewing the fat: The good fat and the good cholesterol." *New England Journal of Medicine* 325 (1991):1740–1741.

Sirtori, C. R., E. Tremoli, E. Gatti, et al. "Controlled evaluation of fat intake in the Mediterranean diet: Comparative activities of olive oil and corn oil on plasma lipids and platelets in high-risk patients." *American Journal of Clinical Nutrition* 44 (1986):635–642.

Stevens, Laura J., et al. "Essential fatty acid metabolism in boys with attention-deficit hyperactivity disorder." *American Journal of Clinical Nutrition* 62 (1995):761 –768.

Trevisan, M., V. Krogh, J. Freudenheim, A. Blake, et al., and the Research Group ATS-RF2 of the Italian National Research Council. "Consumption of olive oil, butter, and vegetable oils and coronary heart disease risk factors." *Journal of the American Medical Association* 263 (1990):688–692.

A FEAST OF HEALTH FROM THE SEA

Albert, C. M., C. H. Hennekens, C. J. O'Donnell, U. A. Ajani, et al. "Fish consumption and risk of sudden cardiac death." *Journal of the American Medical Association* 279 (1998):1, 23–28.

Ascherio, A., E. B. Rimm, M. J. Stampfer, E. L. Giovannucci, et al. "Dietary intake of marine n-3 fatty acids, fish intake, and the risk of coronary disease among men." *New England Journal of Medicine* 332 (1995):977–982.

Broughton, K. Shane, et al. "Reduced asthma symptoms

with n-3 fatty acid ingestion are related to 5-series leukotriene production." *American Journal of Clinical Nutrition* 65 (1997):1011–1017.

Daviglus, M. L., J. Stamler, A. J. Orencia, A. R. Dyer, et al. "Fish consumption and the 30-year risk of fatal myocardial infarction (heart attack)." *New England Journal of Medicine* 336 (1997):1046–1053.

de Lorgeril, M., et al. "Mediterranean alpha-linolenic acid-rich diet in secondary prevention of coronary heart disease." *Lancet* 343 (1994):1454–1459.

Hodge. et al. "Consumption of oily fish and childhood asthma risk." *Medical Journal of Australia* 164 (1996):137–140.

Kromhout, D., E. B. Bosschieter, and C. de Lezenne Coulander. "The inverse relation between fish consumption and 20-year mortality from coronary heart disease." *New England Journal of Medicine* 312 (1985): 1205–1209.

Kromhout, D., E. J. M. Feskens, and C. H. Bowles. "The protective effect of a small amount of fish on coronary heart disease mortality in an elderly population." *International Journal of Epidemiology* 24 (1995):340–345.

Lukin, D. *The Dean Lukin Diet.* Melbourne: Margaret Gee Publishing, 1993.

Mori, T. A., L. J. Beilin, V. Burke, J. Morris, et al. "Interactions between dietary fat, fish, and fish oils and their effects on platelet function in men at risk of cardiovascular disease." *Arteriosclerosis, Thrombosis, and Vascular Biology* 17 (1997):279–286.

Nagata, C., N. Takatsuka, and H. Shimizu. "Soy and fish oil intake and mortality in a Japanese community." *American Journal of Epidemiology* 156(9) (2002):824–831.

Nettleton, J. A. *Omega-3 Fatty Acids and Health.* New York: Chapman & Hall, 1995, 354.

Nordoy, A. "Omega 3-Fatty Acids and Thrombosis." Proceedings of the Scientific Conference on Omega-3 Fatty Acids in Nutrition, Vascular Biology, and Medicine, Houston, Tex, April 17–19, 1994, 221–231.

Shekelle, R. B., L. Missell, O. Paul, A. M. Shryock, et al. "Fish consumption and mortality from coronary heart disease." *New England Journal of Medicine.* 313 (1985):820.

Simopoulos, A. "Omega-3 fatty acids in health and disease and in growth and development." *American Journal of Clinical Nutrition* 54 (1991): 438-463.

Vollset, S. E., I. Heuch, and E. Bjelke. "Fish consumption and mortality from coronary heart disease." *New England Journal of Medicine* 313 (1985):820–821.

PLANT POWER

Adlercreutz, H., et al. "Dietary phytoestrogens and the menopause in Japan." *Lancet* 339 (1992):1233.

Adlercreutz, H., W. Mazur, et al. "Phytoestrogens and prostate disease." *Journal of Nutrition* 130(3) (2000): 658S–659S.

Albertazzi, P., F. Pansini, G. Bonaccorsi, et al. "The effect of dietary soy supplementation on hot flashes." *Obstetrics and Gynecology* 91 (1998):6–11.

Alekel, D. L., A. S. Germain, et al. "Isoflavone-rich soy protein isolate attentuates bone loss in the lumbar spine of perimenopausal women." *American Journal of Clinical Nutrition* 72(3) (2000):844–852.

Ames, B. N., M. K. Shigenaga, and T. M. Hagen. "Oxidants, antioxidants, and the degenerative diseases of aging." *Proceedings of the National Academy of Sciences* 90 (1993):7915–7922.

Anderson, J. W., B. M. Johnstone, and M. E. Cook-Newell. "Meta-analysis of the effects of soy protein intake on serum lipids." *New England Journal of Medicine* 333 (1995):276–282.

Anthony, M. S. "Soy and cardiovascular disease: cholesterol lowering and beyond." *Journal of Nutrition* 130(3) (2000): 662S–663S.

Arjmandi, B. H., R. Birnbaum, N. V. Goyal, et al. "Bone-sparing effect of soy protein in ovarian hormone-deficient rats is related to its isoflavone content." *American Journal of Clinical Nutrition* 68, suppl. (1998):1364S –1368S.

Block, G., B. Patterson, and A. Subar. "Fruit, vegetables and cancer prevention: A review of the epidemiological evidence." *Nutrition and Cancer* 18 (1992):1–29.

Byers, T., and G. Perry. "Dietary carotenes, vitamin C, and vitamin E as protective antioxidants in human cancers." *Annual Review of Nutrition* 12 (1992):139–159.

Craig, W. "Phytochemicals: Guardians of our health." *Journal of the American Dietetic Association* 97(10) (1996): S199–S204.

Dalais, F. S., et al. "The effects of phytoestrogens in post-menopausal women." *Eighth International Congress on the Menopause Symposium*, 1996.

Diaz, M. N., B. Frei, J. A. Vita, and J. F. Keaney Jr. "Antioxidants and atherosclerotic heart disease." *New England Journal of Medicine* 337 (1997):408–416.

American Institute for Cancer Research. "Food, nutrition and the prevention of cancer: a global perspective." World Cancer Research Fund, Washington D.C., 1997.

Gaziano, J. M., J. E. Manson, L. G. Branch, G. A. Colditz, et al. "A prospective study of consumption of caro-tenoids in fruits and vegetables and decreased cardio-vascular mortality in the elderly." *Annals of Epidemiology* 5 (1995):4, 255–260.

Giovanucci, E., A. Ascherio, E. B. Rimm, M. J. Stampfer, et al. "Intake of carotenoids and retinol in relation to risk of prostate cancer." *Journal of the National Cancer Institute* 87 (1995):1767 –1776.

Harvard University. "Getting the Jump on Osteoporosis." *Harvard Women's Health Watch* 3 (January 1996):1.

Kimira, M., et al. "Japanese intake of flavonoids and isofla-vonoids from foods." *Journal of Epidemiology* 3 (1998): 168–175.

Klipstein-Grobusch, K., et al. "Dietary antioxidants and risk of myocardial infarction (heart attack) in the eld-erly: The Rotterdam Study." *American Journal of Clinical Nutrition* 69 (1999):261.

Kohlmier, L., J. D. Kark, E. Gomez-Garcia, C. B. Martin, et al. "Lycopene and myocardial infarction (heart attack) in the EURAMIC Study." *American Journal of Epidemiology* 146 (1997):618–626.

Kotsopoulos, D., F. S. Dalais, et al. "The effects of soy pro-tein containing phytoestrogens on menopausal symp-toms in postmenopausal women." *Climacteric* 3 (2000): 161–167.

Kromhout, D., E. B. Bosschieter, and C. De Lezenne Coulander. "Dietary fibre and 10-year mortality from coronary heart disease, cancer, and all causes." *Lancet* ii (1982):518–522.

Lamartiniere, C. A. "Protection against breast cancer with genistein: A component of soy." *American Journal of Clinical Nutrition* 71, 6 Suppl. (2000): 1705S–1707S; 1708S–1709S.

Lang, S. "China Study shows need for eating plant-based diet." *Cornell Chronicle* 1 (December 1994), http://environlink.org/arrs/essays/vegdiet.html

Lo, G. S., A. P. Goldberg, A. Lim, et al. "Soy fiber improves lipid and carbohydrate metabolism in primary hyper-lipidemic subjects." *Atherosclerosis* 62 (1986):239–248.

Manson, J., et al. "A prospective study of antioxidant vita-mins and incidence of coronary heart disease in women." *Circulation* 84 (1991):4:11–546.

Messina, M., et al. "Soyfoods, soybean isoflavones, and bone health: A brief overview." *Journal of Renal Nutri-tion* 10(2) (2000):63–68.

Pollard, M. and W. Wolter. "Prevention of spontaneous prostate-related cancer in Lobund-Wistar rats by a soy protein isolate/isoflavone diet." *Prostate* 45(2) (2000): 101–105.

Potter, S. M., J. A. Baum, H. Teng, et al. "Soy protein and isoflavones: Their effects on blood lipids and bone den-sity in postmenopausal women." *American Journal of Clinical Nutrition* 68, suppl. (1998):1375S–1379S.

Potter, S. M. "Soy protein and cardiovascular disease: The impact of bioactive components in soy." *Nutrition Reviews* 56 (1998):231–235.

Rimm, E. B., A. Ascherio, E. Giovannucci, D. Spiegelman, M. Stampfer, and W. C. Willett. "Vegetable, fruit and cereal fiber intake and risk of coronary heart disease among men." *Journal of the American Medical Association* 275 (1996):447–451.

Rose, D. "Diet fiber, phytoestrogens, and breast cancer." *Nutrition* Jan–Feb (1992):47–51.

Steinmetz, K. A., and J. D. Potter. "Vegetables, fruit and cancer: Mechanisms." *Cancer Causes and Control* 2 (1991):427–442.

———. "Vegetables, fruit and cancer prevention: A review." *Journal of the American Dietetic Association* 96 (1996):1027–1039.

Tavani, A., E. Negri, B. Davanzo, and C. La Vecchia. "Beta-carotene intake and risk of nonfatal acute myocardial infarction (heart attack) in women." *European Journal of Epidemiology* 13 (1997):6, 631–637.

Tucker, K. L., M. R. Hannan, H. Chen, L. A. Cupples, et al. "Potassium, magnesium, and fruit and vegetable intakes are associated with greater bone mineral densi-ty in elderly men and women." *American Journal of Clinical Nutrition* 69 (1999): 727–736.

de Lorgeril, M., and P. Salen. "Wine ethanol, platelets and Mediterranean diet." *Lancet* 353(9158) (1999):1067.

Farchi, G., et al. "Alcohol and mortality in the Italian rural cohorts of the Seven Countries Study." *International Journal of Epidemiology* 1(1) (1992):74–81.

Heath, D. *International Handbook on Alcohol and Culture.* Westport, CT: Greenwood Press, 1995.

Hendriks, H., et al. "Effect of moderate dose of alcohol with evening meal on fibrinolytic factors." *British Medical Journal* 308 (1994):1003–1006.

Fuhrman, B., et al. "Consumption of red wine with meals reduces the susceptibility of human plasma and low density lipoprotein to lipid peroxidation." *American Journal of Clinical Nutrition* 61 (1995):549–554.

Haas, C. "Barley, the olive and wine, dietary and therapeutic triad of ancient Mediterranean people." *Annales de Medecine Interne* (Paris) 149(5) (1998):275–279.

Kushi, L., et al. "Health implications of Mediterranean diets in light of contemporary knowledge: 2. Meat, wine, fats, and oils." *American Journal of Clinical Nutrition* 61 (1995):1416S–1427S.

———. "Physical activity and mortality in postmenopausal women." *Journal of the American Medical Association* 30 (1997):1287–1292.

Kondo, K., et al. "Inhibition of oxidation of low-density lipoprotein with red wine." *Lancet* 344 (1994):1152–1153.

Rimm, E. B., E. L. Giovannucci, W.C. Willett, G.A. Colditz, et al. "Prospective study of alcohol consumption and risk of coronary disease in men." *Lancet* 331 (1991):464–468.

Goodrick, G. K., and J. P. Foreyt. "Why treatments for obesity don't work." *Journal of the American Dietetic Association* 91(10) (1991):1243–1247.

Gortmaker, S. L., W. H. Dietz, and L. W. Y. Cheubg. "Inactivity, diet and the fattening of America." *Journal of the American Dietetic Association* 90(9) (1990):1247–1255.

Grundy, S. M., and B. P. Barnett. "Metabolic and health complications of obesity." *Disease-a-Month* 36 (1990): 645–696.

Keys, A., C. Aravanis, H. Blackburn, R. Buzina, B. S. Djordjevic, A. S. Dontas, F. Fidanza, et al. *Seven Countries. A Multivariate Analysis of Death and Coronary Heart Disease.* Cambridge, MA: Harvard University Press, 1980.

Paffenbarger, R. S., R. T. Hyde, A. L. Wing, and C. Hsieh. "Physical activity, all-cause mortality, and longevity of college alumni." *New England Journal of Medicine* 314 (1986):615–613.

Fava Bean(s)
  with Artichoke Hearts, Marinated,
    and Olives, 273
  Bulgur Pilaf with Red Peppers, Pine
    Nuts and, 191
  Eggplant, and Olive Stew with Feta,
    182
  Pasta with Arugula, Prosciutto and,
    151
  Puree with Pita Wedges, 272–273
Fennel, in Grilled Vegetables,
    Mediterranean-Style, 222
Feta
  Fava Bean, Eggplant, and Olive Stew
    with, Greek, 182
  in Greek Salad, 253
  in Greek Salad Pita Pockets, 234
  Pizza, Greek, with Chicken,
    Artichokes and, 170
  Shrimp with, Greek, 179
  and Spinach Parcels, 276
Fiber, dietary, 37, 38–39, 48, 52, 53, 55
Fish. See also Anchovy(ies); Salmon; Tuna
  Burgers with Roasted Red Pepper
    and Wasabi Mayonnaise, 226
  Cakes, Thai, with Sweet Chili Sauce,
    274
  Curry, Thai, 177
  Ginger-Steamed, with Stir-Fried
    Vegetables, 164–165
  omega-3 preventive effects of, 26–30
  Parcels, Thai, 221
  Pasta, Seafood, Sublime, 150
  protein in, 31
  Provençal Baked, with Vegetables, 184
  Sardine Toast Topper, 265
  serving ideas, 33–35
  snack ideas, 126
  Vietnamese Baked, 183
  vitamins and minerals in, 32
  weight loss and, 30–31
Fish oil, 29
5-desmethyl sinensetin, 53
Flavonoids, 53
Focaccia with Smoked Salmon and
    Avocado, 232–233
Folate, 37, 51
French Provençal restaurants, meal
    choices in, 105
Frittata, Tuna, Pea, and Corn, 262
Fritters, Corn, Asian-Style, 275
Fruit(s)
  calories in, 48
  citrus, 53
  fiber in, 38

health benefits of, 46–47
intake of, 45–46
Oatmeal, Creamy Nut and, 266
serving ideas, 46
snacks, 126
superfoods, 49–54
Fruit desserts. See also Compote
  Apple and Walnut Pie, Provençal,
    294–295
  Berry Coulis, Mixed, with Greek
    Vanilla Yogurt, 292
  Couscous with Honey-Cinnamon
    Yogurt, 292–293
  Mango with Lime Syrup and Toasted
    Coconut, 293
  Orange, Date, and Pistachio Salad,
    Tunisian, 295
  Pears with Peach Ricotta Whip and
    Almonds, 294
  Salad, Asian-Style, 296
  Salad, Mango, Grape, and Honeydew
    Melon, 297
  Strawberries and Mascarpone Cheese,
    296
Fullness, feeling of, 20

G
Gado Gado, 259
Garlic
  Aioli, 287
  Asparagus with Toasted Almonds and,
    272
  health benefits of, 49
  Shrimp, 270
  and White Bean Soup, Tuscan, 241
Ginger
  Fish, -Steamed, with Stir-Fried
    Vegetables, 164–165
  Honey Sauce, Stir-Fried Scallops and
    Vegetables with, 156
Glaspy, John, 6
Grain foods. See also Bulgur; Couscous;
    Noodle(s); Pasta; Rice
  carbohydrates in, 40–41
  fiber in, 37, 38–39
  health benefits of, 37
  in meal combinations, 96–103
  with protein sources, 39, 41, 56
  types of, 42–44
  white vs whole grain, 41
Grains, types of, 37
Grape, Mango, and Honeydew Melon
    Salad, 297
Greek diet, Westernization of, 15
Greek restaurants, meal choices in, 105

Greek Salad, 253
  Pita Pockets, 234
Green Beans
  in Beef, Stir-Fried, in Black Bean
    Sauce, 162
  in Fish Curry, Thai, 177
  in Fish with Vegetables, Provençal
    Baked, 184
  in Gado Gado, 259
  in Moroccan Stew with Couscous,
    181
  in Pasta Primavera, 145
  Pasta with Tuna, Olives, Romesco
    Sauce and, 154
  in Salade Niçoise, 254
  in Stir-Fried Tofu, Vegetables, and
    Water Chestnuts in Oyster Sauce,
    157
  in Tuna, Olive, and Vegetable Pasta,
    Lemony, 146

H
Ham
  and Chicken Chow Mein in Peking
    Sauce, 197
  and Egg Fried Rice, 194
  Mushroom, and Tomato Pizza, 169
  in Sandwich, Pan-Fried, Italian-Style,
    268
  soy, 60
Harvard School of Public Health, 6, 8
HDL cholesterol, 16, 21, 49, 63
Heart disease prevention
  alcohol consumption in, 63, 64
  Asian diet and, 2–5
  fiber intake and, 38
  fruits and vegetables in, 47, 50
  grain foods in, 37
  Mediterranean diet and, 2–4, 5–6
  nuts in, 60
  omega-3 fatty acids and, 27–28
  physical activity in, 73
  soybeans in, 57
Heart disease risk
  alcohol abuse and, 65
  saturated fat and, 10–13
  stress as, 83
Heaton, Kenneth, 48
Hegsted, Mark, 5
Hensrud, Donald D., 49
Herbert, James, 14–15
High blood pressure, 17, 28, 73
Hippocrates, 44, 49
Hoisin-Sesame Dipping Sauce, 288
Hom, Ken, 49